A Colour Handbook of
Renal
Medicine

JAMES PATTISON DM FRCP
Consultant Nephrologist
Guy's and St Thomas' Hospital, London, UK

DAVID GOLDSMITH FRCP
Consultant Nephrologist
Guy's and St Thomas' Hospital, London, UK

BARRIE HARTLEY FRCPath
Consultant Renal Pathologist
St James' University Hospital, Leeds, UK

FERNANDO C. FERVENZA MD DPhil
Assistant Professor of Medicine
Mayo Clinic, Rochester, Minnesota, USA

JOSEPH P. GRANDE MD PhD
Professor of Laboratory Medicine and Pathology
Mayo Clinic, Rochester, Minnesota, USA

MANSON
PUBLISHING

A CIP catalogue record for this book is available from the British Library.

For full details of all Manson Publishing Ltd titles please write to:
Manson Publishing Ltd, 73 Corringham Road, London NW11 7DL, UK.
Tel: +44(0)20 8905 5150
Fax: +44(0)20 8201 9233
Website: www.manson-publishing.com

Commissioning editor: Jill Northcott
Project manager: Paul Bennett
Copy-editor: Kathryn Rhodes
Designer: Alpha Media
Colour reproduction by Tenon & Polert Colour Scanning Ltd, Hong Kong
Printed in China by New Era Printing Company Ltd

Contents

Preface

Renal medicine is one of modern medicine's great success stories. Although uroscopy is an ancient art, the modern discipline of nephrology owes its development to recent technologic advances. The advent of the ante-mortem renal biopsy in the early part of the last century was fundamental to achieving an understanding of the way the kidney was affected by intrinsic and systemic diseases. As important was the use of micropuncture techniques which unravelled some of the mysteries of renal tubular physiology; while the development in the 1950s and 60s of the mainstays of modern nephrology – dialysis and renal transplantation – depended on technical advances in bio-engineering, anticoagulation, and immunology.

More than any other subdivision of general internal medicine, successful nephrologic practice is dependent on other specialties. This is so for three reasons: first, the expertise needed in renal imaging, arterial intervention and particularly renal histopathologic examination; second, because of the extent to which the kidneys are affected by so many systemic diseases; and third, because of the increased incidence of cardiovascular and neoplastic disease in patients with long-term renal failure.

The format of this book primarily reflects the 'stages' of renal disease – presenting symptoms and syndromes, inherited renal diseases, glomerular and systemic diseases, acute and chronic renal failure, dialysis, and renal transplantation. This is how trainees at the resident and clinical fellow/senior house officer and registrar levels – at whom this book is aimed – will see their patients. A short book of this nature cannot hope to be all-embracing or comprehensive, but we hope that we have covered the main areas of interest and importance. We hope also that we have shown an 'approach' to nephrologic problems which nonrenal specialist trainees will find useful too.

James Pattison
David Goldsmith
Barrie Hartley
Fernando C. Fervenza
Joseph P. Grande

Acknowledgements

We are very grateful to a number of colleagues for providing illustrative material. These include Dr A. Kawashima, Dr B. King, Dr V. Torres, Dr J. McCarthy, Dr P. Harris, Dr G. Miller, Dr D. Milliner, Dr N. Campeau, Dr R. Desnick, Dr J. Berstein, Dr J. Reidy, Dr A. Saunders, Dr J. Bingham, Dr S. Rankin, Dr G. Rottenberg, Dr T. Gibson, Dr I. Abbs, Dr R. Hilton, Dr J. Cunningham, Dr D. Pennell, Dr P. Ackrill, Dr M. Venning, Dr D. Radia, Dr D. Davies, Dr N. Roussak, Dr S. Clarke, Dr P. Hawkins, Dr F. Tungekar, Dr J. Hextall, Dr C. Reid, Mr G. Swana, Dr B. Hunt, Dr R. Swaminathan, Dr R. Palmer, Dr G. Fogazzi, and Mr D. Spalton. We would like to thank Mr Bill Edwards, Keeper of the Gordon Museum, Guy's Hospital for allowing us to reproduce some of the images of specimens from the Museum.

Certain figures (Chapter 5: figures 118–128) are reproduced with permission from Grainger and Allison: *Diagnostic Radiology* (Chapter 67: Renal arteriography, renovascular disorders and renovascular hypertension), Harcourt Health Sciences, London.

Abbreviations

AA secondary amyloidosis.
ACE angiotensin converting enzyme.
ADH antidiuretic hormone.
ADMA asymmetric dimethylarginine.
ADPKD autosomal dominant polycystic kidney disease.
AGT alanine glyoxylate aminotransferase.
AIDS acquired immune deficiency syndrome.
AIN acute interstital nephritis.
AL primary amyloidosis.
ANA anti-nuclear antibodies.
ANCA anti-neutrophil cytoplasmic antibodies.
Ang angiotensin.
anti-Sm anti-Smith antibodies.
anti-Scl anti-scleroderma antibodies.
APD automated peritoneal dialysis.
APS anti-phospholipid antibody syndrome.
ARBs angiotensin receptor blockers.
ARF acute renal failure.
ARPKD autosomal recessive polycystic kidney disease.
AS Alport's syndrome.
ASO antibody to streptolysin O.
ATN acute tubular necrosis.
AV arteriovenous.
AVF arteriovenous fistula.

BFH benign familial hematuria.
BK BK virus.
(S, D) BP (systolic, diastolic) blood pressure.
C3 Nef C3 nephritic factors.
CABG coronary artery bypass graft.
CAD coronary artery disease.
CAPD continuous ambulatory peritoneal dialysis.
CAVH continuous arteriovenous filtration.
CCB calcium channel blockers.
CLL chronic lymphatic leukemia.
CMV cytomegalovirus.
CNS congenital nephrotic syndrome.
CREST cutaneous systemic sclerosis.
CRF chronic renal failure.
CRP c-reactive protein.
CT computerized tomography.
CUA calcific uremic arteriolopathy.
CVVH continuous venovenous hemofiltration.
CVVHDF continuous venovenous hemodiafiltration.
CXR chest X-ray.

DAT direct antigen testing.
DIC disseminated intravascular coagulation.
DMS diffuse mesangial sclerosis.
DMSA dimercaptosuccinate.
(ds) DNA (double stranded) deoxyribonucleic acid.
DSA digital subtraction angiogram.
DTPA diethylenetriamine penta acetate.
DVT deep vein thrombosis.

EKG electrocardiogram.
ECHO echocardiogram.
ECV effective circulating volume.
EDTA ethylene diamine tetra-acetic acid.
ELISA enzyme-linked immunosorbent assay.
ENT ear, nose and throat.
ESR erythrocyte sedimentation rate.
ESRD end-stage renal disease.
ESRF end-stage renal failure.

FFP fresh frozen plasma.
FSGS focal segmental glomerulosclerosis.

Gal galactose.
GalNAc N-acetylgalactosamine.
Gb3 galactotriosylceramide.
GBM glomerular basement membrane.
GFR glomerular filtration rate.
GI gastrointestinal.
GN glomerulonephritis.

HBcAg hepatitis B core antigen.
HBeAg hepatatis B e antigen.
HBsAg hepatitis B surface antigen.
HBV hepatitis B virus.
HCV hepatitis C virus.
HD hemodialysis.
HDL high density lipoprotein.
H+E hematoxylin and eosin stain.
HIF hypoxia-inducible factor.
HIV human immunodeficiency virus.
HIVAN human immunodeficiency virus-associated nephropathy.
HLA human leukocyte antigen.
HUS hemolytic–uremic syndrome.

ICU intensive care unit.
IDNT Irbesartan Diabetic Nephropathy Trial.
Ig (A, G, M) immunoglobulin (A, G, M).
IgAN IgA nephropathy.

INR internal normalized ratio.
IVU intravenous urogram.

JC JC virus.

LDH lactate dehydrogenase.
LDL low density lipoprotein.
LV left ventricle.
LVF left ventricular failure.
LVH left ventricular hypertrophy.

MAP mean arterial pressure.
MCGN mesangiocapillary
    glomerulonephritis.
MCKD medullary cystic kidney disease.
MDRD modification of diet in renal disease.
MN membranous nephropathy.
MPGN membranoproliferative
    glomerulonephritis.
MR magnetic resonance.
MRA magnetic resonance angiography.
MRFIT The Multiple Risk Factor
    Intervention Trial.
MRI magnetic resonance imaging.
MS methenamine silver.

NO nitric oxide.
NPH nephronophthisis.
NS nephrotic syndrome.
NSAID nonsteroidal anti-inflammatory drug.

PAPS primary anti-phospholipid antibody
    syndrome.
PAS periodic acid Schiff.
PCR polymerase chain reaction.
PD peritoneal dialysis.
PDGF-B platelet-derived growth factor B
    chain.
PET positron emission tomography.
PH primary hyperoxalurias.
PKD polycystic kidney disease.
PTFE polytetrafluoroethylene.
PTH parathyroid hormone.
PSGN poststreptococcal glomerulonephritis.
PTLD post-transplant lymphoproliferative
    disease.
PTRA percutaneous transluminal renal
    angioplasty.
PTX parathyroidectomy.
PUJ pelviureteric junction.

RBC red blood cell.
(m)RNA (messenger) ribonucleic acid.
RPF retroperitoneal fibrosis.
RPGN rapidly progressive
    glomerulonephritis.
RRT renal replacement therapy.

RTA renal tubular acidosis.
RVT renal vein thrombosis.

SAA serum amyloid A protein.
SAP serum amyloid P protein.
SLE systemic lupus erythematosus.

TB tuberculosis.
TBM tubular basement membrane.
TGF transforming growth factor.
TINU tubulointerstitial nephritis–uveitis
    syndrome.
TPN total parenteral nutrition.
TSC tuberous sclerosis complex.
TTP thrombotic thrombocytopenic purpura.

USRDS United States Renal Disease Service.

VEGF vascular endothelial growth factor.
VHL von Hippel–Lindau.
VLDL very low density lipoprotein.
VUJ vesicoureteric junction.

WBC white blood cell.
WHO World Health Organization.

Chapter One

Assessment of the patient with renal disease

- **Introduction**

- **Symptoms of renal disease**

- **Physical signs in renal disease**

- **Presenting symptom complexes/syndromes in renal disease**

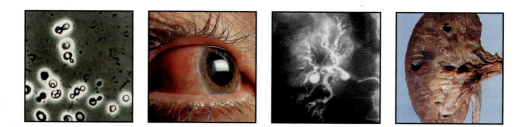

Introduction

Nephrologic problems can first be discovered in the context of acute emergencies with life-threatening potential. More often though the symptoms and signs of more slowly progressive renal disease are occult, subtle, and too often passed off as old age, fatigue, or 'anemia'. There are many thousands of molecules that accumulate in renal failure; ascribing individual symptoms to any one or other of these is unnecessary (and impractical). Many patients on dialysis still have symptoms that first started in the predialysis phase of their illness, as dialysis only replaces about 10% of renal function. Only successful renal transplantation can comprehensively treat the many facets of the uremic syndrome.

Given the major reduction in projected lifespan that ensues with the development of irreversible renal failure, increased emphasis on screening and detection of risk-associations for 'preventable' renal disease, such as raised blood pressure and diabetes, are mandatory.

Renal diseases cover the whole range, from inherited and metabolic/storage derangements to acquired pathologies as diverse as immunologic, metabolic, neoplastic, and infective diseases. Many 'renal' diseases have a systemic component; this is particularly true of immunologic and metabolic problems; the corollary of this is that the first presentation of a problem may well be with symptoms referring to another organ or system. This can lead to misdiagnosis, diagnostic delay, and potential harm, e.g. a patient with epistaxis and nasal blockage may only see a generalist, or an ENT specialist, so that the eventual diagnosis of Wegener's granulomatosis comes to light only after an episode of acute renal failure has ensued.

Screening for renal problems is in the main relatively easily accomplished without invasive investigation. Use of urine testing apparatus to detect the presence of blood and protein in the urine is cheap, fast, and sensitive. Equally, the main blood marker of renal function, serum creatinine concentration, is a part of every biochemical automated analytical profile.

Symptoms of renal disease

ASYMPTOMATIC PATIENTS
Asymptomatic patients are typically detected after routine screening of urine, of blood pressure, and of excretory renal function. This is often after a patient has moved and registered with a new doctor and undergoes health screening, or in the context of a work/insurance medical examination. Other situations include screening during pregnancy, screening due to work-related exposure to renal toxins, or after another family member has been diagnosed with an hereditable renal condition (e.g. polycystic kidney disease).

TIREDNESS
By its very nature this is a symptom that has many different causes. Most patients with significant renal impairment are tired. Anemia, now treated with erythropoietin, was the major reason for this symptom, but many patients report reduced energy levels even with normal hemoglobin concentrations. Hypoalbuminemia is also associated with significant tiredness once plasma albumin has fallen to <30 g/l (<3g/dl).

ITCHING (PRURITUS)
By the time GFR has fallen to <20 ml/min, many patients notice dry skin (xerosis) and itching. This is worse at night, when there is vasodilatation. It is multifactorial, involving altered dermal sensation, opioid metabolism, and calcium–phosphate precipitation. Repeated scratching and excoriation leads to a self-perpetuating cycle of dryness and irritation. Iron deficiency may exacerbate the problem. Rarely nodular prurigo is a feature. Symptomatic relief can be obtained from menthol creams and unguents, from regular moisturizers, from antihistamines, and in some cases, naloxone and other opioid partial agonists (1).

BREATHLESSNESS
Any one of anemia, fluid retention (pulmonary edema, pleural effusions), and acidosis can produce this symptom.

DISTURBED URINARY HABIT (POLYURIA, NOCTURIA, ENURESIS, OLIGURIA, ANURIA)
Polyuria may be due to:
- Increased water intake (e.g. compulsive polydipsia).
- Increase in osmotic load (e.g. urea in chronic renal failure, glucose in diabetes mellitus).
- Reduced ADH secretion (e.g. head injury and central diabetes insipidus).

- Renal resistance to ADH (e.g. inherited nephrogenic diabetes insipidus).
- Acquired conditions (e.g. hypokalemia, hypercalcemia, lithium toxicity).
- Reduced medullary concentrating ability (e.g. interstitial nephritis, papillary necrosis, nephrocalcinosis).

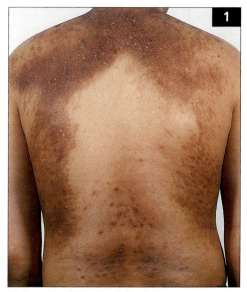

1 View of a CRF patient's back showing a large area (accessible to scratching) of increased pigmentation and excoriation due to uremic pruritus.

Polyuria is seen in the recovery phase of oliguric acute renal failure, after renal transplantation, and after successful angioplasty of a tight renal artery stenosis in a single well-functioning kidney.

Loss of urinary concentrating (distal tubule and collecting system) ability in chronic renal failure, due to loss of functional nephrons and refractoriness of the remnant nephrons to ADH, is manifest by the failure of the normal physiologic mechanisms of decreasing urinary volume and increasing urinary concentration; this leads to nocturia. More observant patients may notice that their urine is clearer, and paler, and uniformly so, i.e. without any diurnal variation. As renal function deteriorates nocturia worsens; many patients need to get up three or four times at night. Urinary stream, and bladder function, are unaffected (symptomatic enquiries on this point are crucial, as prostate and bladder problems also of course have nocturia as part of their symptom complexes). Nocturia, and reversed day–night urine volume excretion, can be seen in the elderly (most probably due to progressive renal impairment), in diabetes mellitus and insipidus, and in hypothyroidism.

Oliguria (less than 400 ml urine/24 h) is a feature of acute renal failure (though many such cases of ARF have a transient oliguric phase). Anuria is usually due to complete urinary tract obstruction (2–4) though more rarely seen with acute cortical necrosis, or bilateral renal infarction.

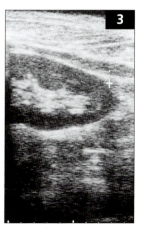

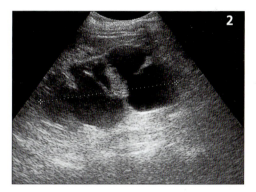

2 Renal tract ultrasound showing gross hydronephrosis and renal cortical thinning in a case of obstructive uropathy.

3 Renal tract ultrasound showing normal appearance with compact echogenic pelvis and clear cortico-medullary differentiation.

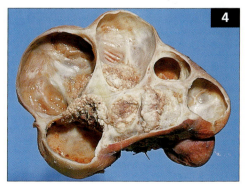

4 Postmortem appearance of chronic severe hydronephrosis. Note the virtual absence of renal cortex.

Symptoms of renal disease (*continued*)

BLOOD IN URINE (HEMATURIA)

Macroscopic hematuria (**5**) can be one of the most alarming symptoms from a patient's perspective. Pink/red/brown urine can also be seen with anthocyanin ingestion (e.g. beetroot), rhabdomyolysis, porphyria, alkaptonuria, rifampin (rifampicin) or phenytoin therapy, and after phenolphthalein ingestion. Very rarely it can be factitious (e.g. nucleated red blood cells seen on urine microscopy after a patient persistently 'spiked' her urine with chicken blood!).

In healthy subjects $<10^7$ red blood cells (RBCs) are excreted in the urine per day. This equates approximately to one erythrocyte per microliter of urine. Only 5 ml of blood containing 25×10^9 RBCs in one liter of urine is needed to give macroscopic hematuria. Hematuria can be microscopic only, macroscopic only, or intermittent macroscopic with persistent microscopic. Blood can of course arise from anywhere in the urinary tract. Hemoglobinopathies such as sickle cell disease (and trait) are associated with microscopic hematuria. Jogging and heavy physical exercise often cause transient microscopic hematuria.

Urinary testing using dipstick reagents is convenient and practical at home and in hospital settings. These reagents detect the hemoglobin from lysed RBCs. The sensitivity of these tests is high, and close to the normal RBC excretion rate. Microscopy of urine is best done with freshly-voided acid urine (e.g. first voided after overnight recumbency) as this avoids premature breaking-up of the cell membranes. Sometimes renal hematuria can be so heavy that clots are seen. *Table 1* lists the major causes of hematuria.

Red blood cells that have traversed Bowman's space and the tubular system in the nephron characteristically have abnormal shapes compared to those that arise from lower urinary tract bleeding – so called 'dysmorphic' RBCs. These can be recognized in freshly-voided urine by means of urinary centrifugation and phase-contrast microscopy (**6, 7**). Red cells trapped in hyaline-proteinaceous casts in the urine – red cell casts – are a cardinal sign of acute glomerulonephritis (**8**).

PROTEINURIA

This has become a common presentation for patients with renal disease in the era of urine screening using stick reagents.

Conditions such as hypertension and diabetes in which there is glomerular hypertension (thereby altering glomerular permeability) are often associated with the development of glomerular proteinuria.

Certain groups, such as diabetics and hypertensives, will have their urine checked regularly for protein (in fact for albumin as micro-albuminuria, or albumin excretion rate, or albumin/creatinine ratio). The development and persistence of this urinary abnormality immediately raises the mortality risk of the individual (as much due to cardiovascular disease as malign renal outcome).

Protein in the urine can be glomerular or tubular in origin. Protein is virtually excluded 100% from glomerular filtrate due to poorly understood mechanisms that include pore size, permselectivity of the renal basement membrane, and cell membrane charge. Normal protein

---

Table 1 Renal causes of hematuria

Coagulopathies
Anticoagulants
Hemophilia, sickle

Glomerular disease
IgA nephropathy
Alport's syndrome
Thin membrane disease
Systemic vasculitis/lupus
MCGN/RPGN

Tumors
Renal cell carcinoma
Transitional cell carcinoma

Stones
Anywhere in urinary tract
Calcium oxalate, urate

Medullary/interstitial disease
Papillary necrosis
Medullary sponge kidney
Tuberculosis

Traumatic
Kidney, ureter

Miscellaneous
Hereditary hemorrhagic telangiectasia
Arteriovenous malformations
Loin-pain hematuria

excretion is about 100 mg protein/day; over half of this is albumin. The upper limit of normal for protein excretion is taken as 150 mg/day. Experimental data suggest a heteroporous model to explain the development of proteinuria in renal disease – the development of more membrane pores, and the appearance of larger membrane pores. Glomerular proteinuria can be anything from 0.2–100 g/24 h.

Tubules can actively reabsorb protein. Greater than 95% of low molecular weight filtered proteins are reabsorbed in the proximal tubule. Proximal tubular damage will give rise to 'tubular proteinuria' which is rarely >1 g/24 h.

Beta-2-microglobulin, and Tamm–Horsfall protein (secreted, and a major component of renal tubular casts), are two main constituents of tubular proteinuria.

Cardiac failure, heavy exercise, and orthostatic proteinuria all need careful confirmation or exclusion. Young males seem most prone to supine/orthostatic proteinuria (not completely understood but perhaps an exaggerated glomerular hemodynamic response to change in posture). This condition appears to be benign.

A renal biopsy is indicated if there is >1 g of protein loss/24 h or there is evidence of renal impairment or progressive loss of renal function.

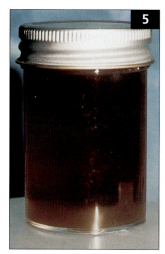

5 A pot of urine showing gross macroscopic hematuria.

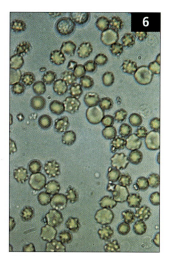

6 Urine microscopy showing normal red blood cells in the urine.

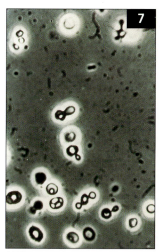

7 Phase contrast urine microscopy showing cells which have irregular not smooth outlines and are 'dysmorphic'.

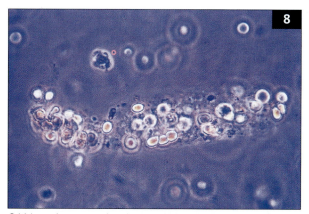

8 Urine microscopy showing a red blood cell cast (red blood cells in the urine trapped in a hyaline cast).

Symptoms of renal disease (*continued*)

SWELLING (EDEMA)

Salt and water retention is one of the early manifestations of the acute or chronic loss of functional nephrons. This produces symptoms and signs depending on the location of the fluid. Edema is most often first noticed as periorbital puffiness on rising, and ankle edema at the end of the day (**9, 10**). It is of fundamental importance to understand whether edema is due to local factors (e.g. vasodilatation or poor venous drainage), or to systemic causes such as cardiac or renal failure, or hypoalbuminemia. Testing the urine for the presence of blood and protein is a cardinal investigation of edema, and should certainly precede the prescription of a diuretic.

Ascites, pleural, and pericardial effusions (**11**) can accompany severe edema such as seen in advanced nephrotic syndrome.

LOSS OF APPETITE (ANOREXIA, NAUSEA)

With advanced renal failure come anorexia, nausea, and eventually vomiting. Acidemia is anorectic and catabolic. Leptin retention may play a role in anorexia; while 'middle molecules' are associated with the gastrointestinal symptoms. Well dialysed patients tend to eat better than poorly dialysed ones, and aggressive treatment of renal anemia can also improve appetite.

TWITCHING/RESTLESS LEGS (MYOCLONUS)/NUMBNESS–BURNING (PAR- OR DYSESTHESIA)

Middle molecule retention in advanced chronic renal failure, or on dialysis, can lead to painful peripheral (mainly sensory but sometimes motor or autonomic) neuropathy. Myoclonic jerks (restless legs) are a typical symptom, sometimes also associated with sleep disturbance or sleep apnea, in advanced chronic renal failure or on dialysis. Clonazepam, diazepam, phenytoin, and gabapentin have all been tried with some success. Initiating dialysis, or improving solute clearance on dialysis, may help, but the definitive treatment remains renal transplantation.

LOIN PAIN

This is an inconsistent accompaniment to renal diseases. Patients often describe back and loin pain but mechanical back problems are more commonly the cause. Acute pyelonephritis is often painful; renal vein thrombosis rarely so. Acute IgA nephropathy and poststreptococcal glomerulonephritis can be associated with loin aching, especially if there is significant macroscopic hematuria.

IMPORTANT FACETS OF THE HISTORY IN RENAL DISEASE

- Previous estimations of BP, urine testing, and renal function testing.
- Childhood problems (e.g. enuresis, recurrent fevers).
- Drug history (prescribed, borrowed, 'over-the-counter', illicit).
- Gynecological and obstetric history.
- Family history.
- Occupational and social histories.
- Travel history.

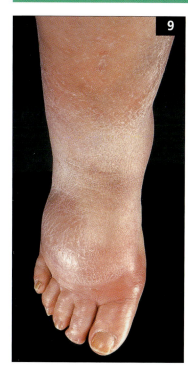

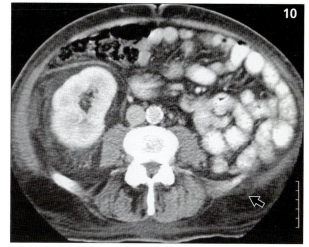

10 Abdominal CT scan showing massive sacral edema (arrow).

9 Gross edema of the lower leg in nephrotic syndrome.

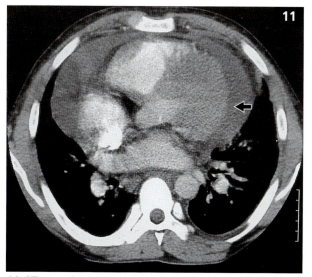

11 CT scan of the chest showing a large pericardial effusion (arrow).

Physical signs in renal disease

A full physical examination is an essential part of a proper nephrologic diagnosis. Leuconychia indicates chronic ill-health; a pigmented band at the distal edge of the nail indicates chronic uremia (**12**).

Inspection of the kidneys is rarely rewarding, though occasional patients of slim physique and with large polycystic kidneys may have obvious abdominal distention (**13**).

Palpation of the lower pole of the right kidney in full inspiration in a slim individual is a normal finding. Polycystic kidneys, large solitary lower pole cysts, and malignant tumors can all be palpated on occasions.

General physical examination is important where renal pathology has affected other organs and systems, or in the context of a multisystem disease. Thus, purpura can manifest Henoch–Schöenlein purpura (**14, 15**), or vasculitis; butterfly rash and nail-fold infarcts can reveal systemic lupus erythematosus (**16**); periumbilical and genital pigmented hyperkeratotic papules are seen in Fabry's disease (**17**); peripalpebral purpura (**18**) is a feature of extensive amyloidosis; partial lipodystrophy (**19**) is most often associated with mesangiocapillary glomerulonephritis. Scleroderma has a characteristic appearance of the face and hands (**20, 134, 135**).

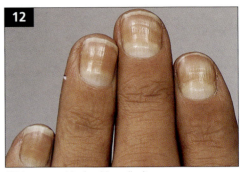

12 Leuconychia (and jaundice).

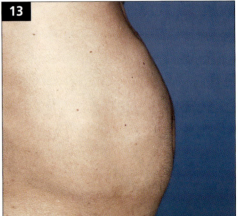

13 Central abdominal swelling due to the presence of grossly enlarged polycystic kidneys in a case of autosomal dominant polycystic kidney disease.

14, 15 Low power view of the buttocks and extensor surface of the legs (**14**). A widespread 'vasculitic' rash is present. Higher power view of individual lesions (**15**).

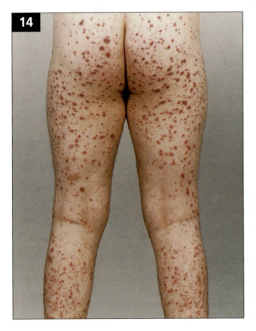

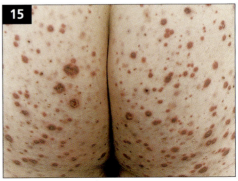

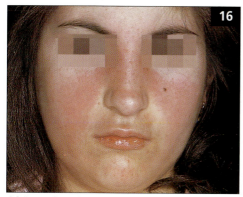

16 Butterfly rash in a patient with SLE.

17 Characteristic dermatological appearance (angiokeratoma corporis diffusum universale) of Fabry's disease in a transplanted patient. The lesions are typically in a bathing trunk distribution. The hirsutism reflects cyclosporine (cyclosporin) treatment.

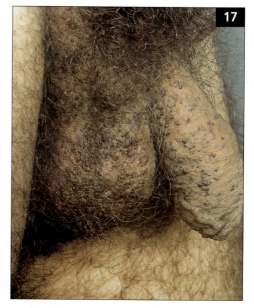

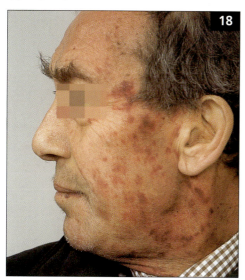

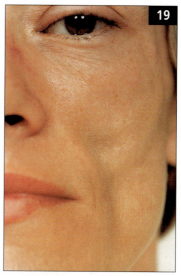

18 Spontaneous peri-orbital palpebral (and facial) purpura on the neck, due to skin chaffing from a shirt-collar. Extensive skin amyloidosis renders skin capillaries very fragile.

19 Partial lipodystrophy in a patient with mesangiocapillary glomerulonephritis. Partial lipodystrophy is also seen spontaneously, in families, and in the context of antiviral therapy in some HIV-positive patients.

20 Scleroderma producing swollen red featureless fingers with 'tight' skin.

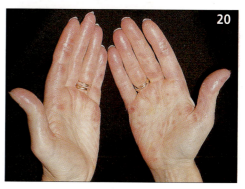

Physical signs in renal disease (*continued*)

Finger infarction, iritis, and collapse of the nasal cartilage (**21–23**) heralds Wegener's granulomatosis.

Examination of the eye can lead to helpful clues – hypercalcemia induces limbal calcification and redness (**24**); vasculitis and sarcoidosis are associated with uveitis and episcleritis; Alport's syndrome is associated with lenticonus (**194**); nephronophthisis with tapetoretinal degeneration (Senior–Loken syndrome) (**192**).

Fundoscopy is crucial to the diagnosis and evaluation of hypertension and diabetes (**25**). Gross neuropathic muscle wasting is seen in severe mononeuritis multiplex in diabetes (**26**).

Sometimes a single investigation will yield an immediate diagnostic answer. Obviously this applies to renal biopsy. Renal angiography can also reveal a reason for renal problems, including multiple microaneurysms of the renal arterial branches in classic polyarteritis nodosa (**27**).

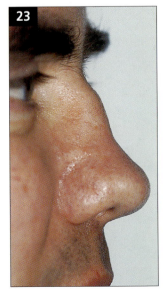

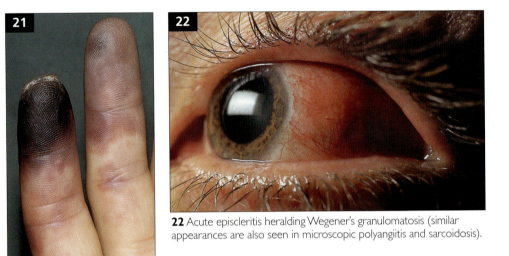

22 Acute episcleritis heralding Wegener's granulomatosis (similar appearances are also seen in microscopic polyangiitis and sarcoidosis).

21 Acute infarction of a digit (a very wide differential diagnosis).

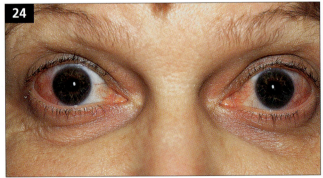

24 Acute red eye of uremia. First described in the 1960s, this is due to ectopic calcification (calcium–phosphate) in the corneal limbus leading to local irritation.

23 Collapse of the nasal cartilage seen in Wegener's granulomatosis (and also in lethal medline granuloma, relapsing polychondritis, and congenital syphilis).

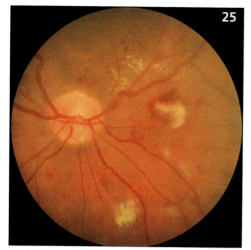

25 Gross proliferative diabetic retinopathy. In type 1 diabetic patients this complication (and neuropathy) is often seen in the context of diabetic nephropathy.

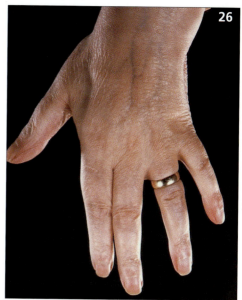

26 Severe muscle wasting due to mononeuritis multiplex in a poorly-controlled diabetic patient.

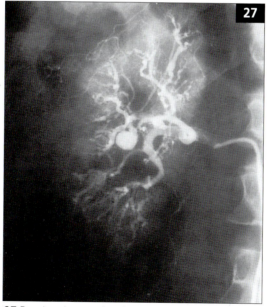

27 Renal angiogram showing multiple micro-aneurysms ('beads') on renal artery branches in a case of classic polyarteritis nodosa.

Presenting symptom complexes/syndromes in renal disease

NEPHROTIC SYNDROME (NS)

This is one of the best known manifestations of renal disease. Its management encapsulates many facets of the care of patients with renal problems. If proteinuria is sufficiently severe and prolonged, nephrotic syndrome (proteinuric, hypoproteinemic edema) will develop.

A good working definition is edema, plasma albumin <30 g/l (3 g/dl) and >3 g of urinary protein loss/24 h. Edema (**9**) can be subtle, or so severe as to be debilitating (anasarca). Nephrotic syndrome is not benign, unless the underlying cause can be treated and the syndrome brought into remission. Patients notice frothy urine in heavy proteinuria (**28**).

Pathogenesis

How edema develops in NS remains controversial. The old classic theory of underfilling due to reduced plasma oncotic pressure is not supported by many more recent careful investigations. Plasmapheresis, which reduces plasma albumin substantially, does not induce edema. Plasma volume measurements usually show normality or even increase, rather than decrease. Sodium and water retention is somehow a concomitant of increased renal tubular protein traffic.

Clinical features

Up to 4 liters of salt and water can remain clinically undetectable. Edema usually starts periorbitally, and can end up being severe with the patient 20 or more kilograms overloaded. Gross pitting skin-splitting lower leg edema, sacral and genital edema, pleural and pericardial effusions, and ascites can all be present in severe cases.

Hyperlipidemia is a typical concomitant and in established persistent NS eruptive xanthomata (**29**) can rarely be seen.

There are very many causes of NS (*Table 2*). To distinguish these a renal biopsy is almost always indicated (the exception being children aged <10 years, in whom a trial of steroids is preferable, reserving biopsy for more problematic management cases).

Complications of nephrotic syndrome

NS can affect many other parts of the body, just as uremia does. Together with the loss of albumin there is usually gross hepatic over-production of many other proteins (not always albumin itself for obscure reasons).

Infections

Bacterial infections are more common in NS and can be life-threatening. This is especially so in adults with NS. Primary peritonitis (often *Streptococcus pneumoniae*, but also gram-negatives and *Hemophilus* spp.) may present insidiously with mild abdominal colicky pain, or with circulatory collapse. Cellulitis arising from skin splits or punctures are a risk in severely edematous limbs. Viral infections may actually trigger relapses in childhood NS due to minimal change nephropathy.

Reasons for increased susceptibility to infection, apart from the physical effects of edema, include hypogammaglobulinemia (reduced IgG), reduced complement (factor B) system activity, low zinc levels, and impaired T-lymphocyte function.

Antibiotic and vaccine prophylaxis seem sensible measures, but rigorous evidence supporting their use is lacking.

Thromboembolic disease

Thrombosis, both venous and arterial, commonly affects severely nephrotic adults (10%) and children (2%); these problems are another reason for the occasional fatalities seen in NS.

There are very many abnormalities in coagulation described in NS. Prothrombotic changes include increases in Von Willebrand factor, fibrinogen, factor V, and protein C. Fibrinolysis is also inhibited. Platelets are reported to be hypercoagulable. Patients with NS can be relatively immobile. Whole blood viscosity may be increased by hyperfibrinogenemia, by diuretics, and perhaps by steroids. The most common site for thrombosis is the deep venous system of the lower limbs; this may go undetected in warm edematous legs until a pulmonary embolus ensues. Renal vein thrombosis (RVT) is seen rarely, though it is thought to be more common in idiopathic and lupus membranous disease, and also in amyloidosis.

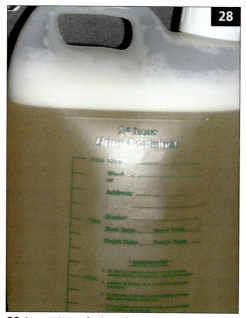

28 A container of urine with an impressive 'head' of froth. Protein in the urine significantly lowers the surface tension of urine and with aeration leads to bubbles. Patients often notice this frothing (which can be mimicked by toilet cleansers).

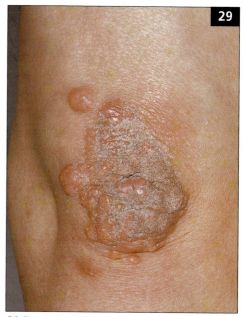

29 Eruptive xanthomata in a nephrotic patient with gross secondary hypercholesterolemia.

Table 2 Common causes of nephrotic syndrome

Primary glomerular
Minimal change
Mesangioproliferative, e.g. IgA
Membranoproliferative
Membranous
Focal and segmental glomerulosclerosis

Secondary glomerular
Diabetes mellitus
Amyloidosis
Systemic lupus erythematosus
HIV-associated nephropathy
Hepatitis C-associated nephropathy

Drugs
Gold
Penicillamine
NSAIDs

Miscellaneous

Presenting symptom complexes/syndromes in renal disease (*continued*)

The extent and severity of venous thromboses will depend on the investigative rigour and zeal employed. In some series RVT can be found in 10% of NS subjects (**30, 31**). The classical presentation of flank pain, deterioration of renal function, macroscopic hematuria, and ipsilateral testicular swelling is as rare as it is well-remembered. Whether it is preferable to seek out the presence of RVT/DVT (using MR venography, CT scanning, or contrast venography), as opposed to taking prophylactic measures for all cases of NS, remains to be established.

Arterial thrombosis is very much rarer in NS but is reported, and can be devastating. The femoral artery is the most commonly reported site (especially in children), but cases have been reported for virtually every artery (**32**).

Treatment and prophylaxis are widely practised, though the evidence-base is slender. Heparin (larger doses are required in NS) and warfarin are the therapeutic mainstays, as well as minimizing hemoconcentration, treating sepsis promptly, and encouraging mobility. The real problems lie in deciding whom to anticoagulate, at what point in their NS, and for how long. Many authorities would advocate the use of warfarin if plasma albumin falls to <25 g/l (2.5 g/dl), particularly with extensive edema. Low molecular weight heparin, aspirin, clopidogrel, and dipyridamole are also (weaker) alternatives.

Dyslipidemia
There is often a severe secondary dyslipidemia in NS. Whether or not this contributes to increased cardiovascular mortality or progressive renal damage in NS is uncertain, but substantial sustained elevations in plasma cholesterol should not be viewed with equanimity. Free cholesterol, cholesterol esters, and phospholipids all increase in NS. Triglycerides can also be elevated. LDL and VLDL concentrations are increased; HDL concentrations are often normal or low. Lipoprotein (a) is also increased. Lipiduria is often a feature of NS.

The reasons for the dyslipidemia remain to be fully elucidated but seem to include a major increase in production and reduction in removal of lipoproteins. There is hugely increased hepatic lipoprotein synthesis in rough proportion to protein loss and hypoalbuminemia. Levels of important lipid regulating enzymes such as lipoprotein lipase and lecithin cholesterol acyl transferase are also deranged in NS.

Treatment can be effective using low-fat diets, statins, and fibrates. Reducing proteinuria (by whatever means) is also helpful to the dyslipidemia.

Loss of binding transport proteins in the urine
Low concentrations of copper, zinc, and iron have been noted in NS plasma. The relevant binding proteins may be lost in the urine. Vitamin D concentrations can also be low in NS. Bone disease may be more common in children with protracted NS. Changes in thyroid-binding globulin and cortisol-binding protein are clinically unimportant.

Catabolism and poor nutrition
Wasting of muscle is a major problem in severe NS. Albumin turnover is greatly increased. The optimal protein intake in NS remains controversial. Cases can be made for normal or high protein diets.

Acute renal failure
This is a rare sequela of NS, and can happen spontaneously when NS is very severe, or after excessive diuresis with loop diuretics.

Treatment of nephrotic syndrome
First and foremost is the need to establish the underlying causation of the NS by means of a careful and thorough history and then a renal biopsy. Where there is a remediable lesion, such as minimal change disease, then immuno-modulatory treatment might induce a remission in days. Many cases of membranous nephropathy can remit spontaneously, or after prednisolone and chlorambucil/cyclophosphamide. In other cases though there is much less likelihood of significant remission, e.g. focal and segmental glomerulosclerosis, or amyloidosis.

Sodium restriction (50 mmol/24 h [50 mEq/24h]) and diuretics will help the edema resolve. Furosemide (frusemide) by mouth may be ineffective as protein binding in the convoluted tubule may prevent its action. Thiazides are synergistic with loop diuretics in this situation. Salt-poor albumin has been widely employed in severe or diuretic-refractory, cases.

Reduction of proteinuria is the goal of therapy. Leaving aside interventions to remove the cause of NS, there are several general measures that can be employed to reduce proteinuria. Most if not all depend on reducing

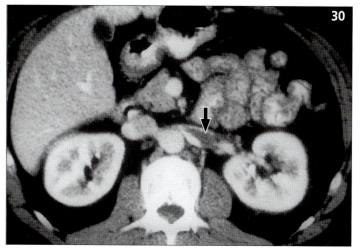

30 CT scan at the level of the kidneys showing a large blood clot in the renal vein (arrow). RVT occurs more often in membranous nephropathy and amyloidosis than in other causes of NS. Loin pain, hematuria, and renal impairment are classic symptoms for a large acute thrombosis; pulmonary emboli are not uncommon.

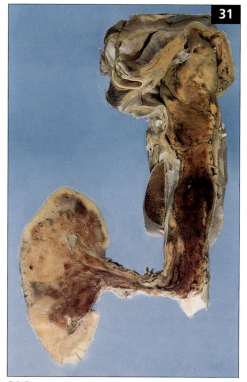

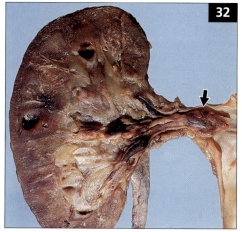

32 Postmortem specimen of acute renal arterial thrombosis (arrow).

31 Postmortem specimen of an acute RVT in a patient with renal amyloidosis (pale kidney) and nephrotic syndrome.

Presenting symptom complexes/syndromes in renal disease (*continued*)

GFR. Older measures included the use of high-dose nonsteroidal anti-inflammatory drugs (often indomethacin), dipyridamole, or cyclosporine (cyclosporin) (which can be an immunomodulatory intervention in its own right in, e.g. steroid-resistant minimal change nephropathy, or membranous glomerulopathy). NSAIDs work rapidly, but have a considerable number of unwelcome side-effects.

Use of the ACE inhibitors, alone, or in concert with angiotensin antagonists, are the modern approach to proteinuria reduction. The dose response curve for proteinuria reduction is different to that of blood pressure reduction; very high doses of these drugs can be used with success. It may take many weeks for the full effect of these drugs to be manifest. Sodium restriction potentiates the antiproteinuric effect of these drugs, as it does for their antihypertensive effect. It is possible to combine say NSAIDs with ACE inhibitors to try to induce an even larger fall in GFR.

Most rarely in adults, and very rarely in children, NS remains severe and patients can fail to thrive, or succumb to complications. If the patients are refractory to several interventions and severely incapacitated by NS, then a single, or double, native nephrectomy can be undertaken. The rationale is the subsequent restoration of plasma albumin by supplementation, of fluid volume control by dialysis, and then renal transplantation. Embolization of the kidneys is another approach to the same goal.

UREMIC SYNDROME

Uremia can be associated with many or few symptoms, depending on its severity and speed of onset. The loss of excretory renal function will be manifest as fluid retention, hypertension, and hyperkalemic acidosis. Plasma calcium may fall and phosphate rise.

Tiredness and lack of physical stamina are typical – only partly explained by anemia. Loss of mental sharpness is insidious (but commented on by some patients once renal function is restored). With severe uremia, confusion, obtundation, seizures, and coma are possible.

Anorexia and nausea, with vomiting when severe, are associated with catabolism and loss of muscle bulk; loss of body substance (weight) may be masked by fluid retention.

Bone pain and myopathy can be seen if renal bone pathology is present (most typically secondary hyperparathyroidism).

These features will be covered in later chapters on acute renal failure, chronic renal failure, and dialysis.

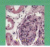
Primary glomerular diseases

- **Minimal change nephropathy**

- **Focal segmental glomerulosclerosis (FSGS)**

- **Thin basement membrane nephropathy**

- **Membranous nephropathy**

- **Membranoproliferative glomerulonephritis (MPGN)**

- **Poststreptococcal glomerulonephritis (PSGN)**

- **IgA nephropathy**

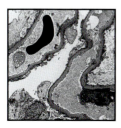
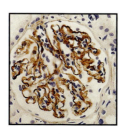
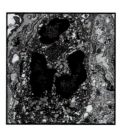
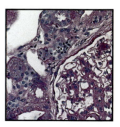

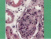

Minimal change nephropathy

DEFINITION
Minimal change nephropathy is defined by the absence of structural glomerular abnormalities other than the presence of epithelial cell foot process fusion on electron microscopy in a patient with proteinuria.

EPIDEMIOLOGY AND ETIOLOGY
It is the most common cause of nephrotic syndrome in children. It is the cause of nephrotic syndrome in 70–90% of cases in children under the age of 10 years, although it rarely occurs before the first year of life. In adolescents and young adults, it is responsible for about 50% cases of nephrotic syndrome, and in older adults about 10–15% of cases.

There is geographic variation in the incidence of minimal change nephropathy, with the disease being more common in Asia than in North America or Europe. It is rare in African-Americans.

PATHOGENESIS
It has been postulated that minimal change nephropathy results from a toxic epithelial cell injury, which results in foot process fusion and detachment of epithelial cells, with disruption of the filtration barrier. The recognition that the disease often remits in children who contract measles, and the association with Hodgkin's lymphoma, suggests that abnormalities in cell-mediated immunity, particularly T-lymphocytes, are involved in pathogenesis, with T-cells producing a lymphokine that increases glomerular permeability to protein. In a minority of patients, there is a clear association with drugs, allergy and malignancy.

CLINICAL HISTORY/PHYSICAL EXAMINATION
The cardinal clinical features in children are: abrupt onset of nephrotic syndrome, manifested by edema, with heavy proteinuria, hypoalbuminemia, and hyperlipidemia. The presence of hematuria, hypertension, or impaired renal function is unusual in children. In adults, hypertension and renal insufficiency are more common.

DIFFERENTIAL DIAGNOSIS
In children, the presence of nephrotic syndrome without microscopic hematuria suggests minimal change nephropathy until proven otherwise. In children who fail to respond to steroids a renal biopsy is justified. In children aged <2 years, congenital nephrotic syndrome and diffuse mesangial sclerosis are important differential diagnoses. In adults, minimal change nephropathy accounts for <30% of the cases of patients presenting with a nephrotic syndrome, and a renal biopsy is required to establish the diagnosis. The most important differential diagnoses are focal segmental glomerulosclerosis (FSGS) and membranous nephropathy. In some patients, minimal change nephropathy may have a secondary cause (*Table 3*).

INVESTIGATIONS
There is usually nephrotic range proteinuria (>3.5g/24 h in adults or $\geq$40 mg/h/m^2 in children) and a low serum albumin. The ESR is raised as a consequence of hyperfibrinogenemia and hypoalbuminemia. There are elevated total cholesterol, LDL, and triglyceride levels. Serum IgG and IgA levels may be reduced, while serum IgM levels can be mildly increased.

Urinalysis is usually normal. A few patients (<15%) may have microscopic hematuria. Under polarized light, oval fat bodies appear as 'Maltese crosses'.

Table 3 Secondary causes of minimal change nephropathy

Infections
Viral (mononucleosis, HIV), parasitic

Drugs
NSAID, gold, lithium, interferon alpha, ampicillin, rifampin (rifampicin), trimethadione

Tumors
Hodgkin's lymphoma, leukemia, solid tumors

Allergies
Food, dust, bee stings, pollen, poison ivy and poison oak

Dermatitis herpetiformis

HISTOLOGY

Light microscopy (33)

By definition there are no glomerular lesions, or only minimal mesangial prominence. The tubules may show lipid droplet accumulation from absorbed lipoproteins. Occasionally, findings consistent with acute tubular necrosis can be seen.

Immunofluorescence microscopy

There is no staining with antisera specific for IgG, IgA, and complement C3, C4, or C1q. In same cases, mesangial IgM is present, although these cases may represent a different entity.

Electron microscopy (34)

Effacement of visceral epithelial cell foot process is the only abnormality. However, this is a nonspecific finding and can be seen in patients with heavy proteinuria secondary to other glomerulopathies.

PROGNOSIS

The overall prognosis is excellent, with patients maintaining renal function long term. The major morbidity of minimal change nephropathy is related to side-effects of therapy. In patients who failed to respond to therapy or who develop progressive renal failure, an alternative diagnosis (such as FSGS) must be considered.

MANAGEMENT

In children, high-dose steroids are the cornerstone of treatment, with >90% of children going into complete remission after 4–6 weeks of treatment. In adolescents and adults, the response to therapy is still high (>80%), but in these age groups the response is slower and some patients may require up to 16 weeks of high-dose steroid use before remission is achieved. Of the patients who respond to steroid therapy, 25% will have a long-term remission. The remaining patients will have at least one or more relapses. For patients who have frequent relapses or are resistant to steroids, alternative therapy includes the use of cyclophosphamide, chlorambucil, mycophenolate mofetil, levamisole, cyclosporine (cyclosporin A), and tacrolimus. More recently deflazacort, an oxazoline derivative of prednisolone but with a lower incidence of side-effects, has shown promise. During relapses supportive treatment of the nephrotic syndrome should be given – diuretics, anticoagulation, and lipid-lowering agents may be necessary.

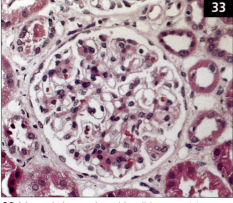

33 Normal glomerulus with mild mesangial prominence. Light microscopy (H+E ×400).

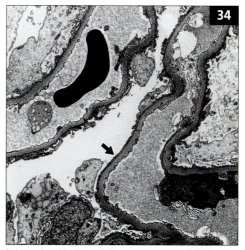

34 Electron microscopy showing diffuse effacement of visceral epithelial cell foot processes (×3400). A continuous band of cytoplasm on the outer aspect of the basement membrane is seen (arrow).

Focal segmental glomerulosclerosis (FSGS)

DEFINITION
FSGS is a diagnostic term for a clinical–pathologic syndrome with multiple etiologies and pathogenic mechanisms. The ubiquitous clinical finding is nephrotic or non-nephrotic proteinuria, and the ubiquitous pathologic feature is focal segmental glomerular consolidation and scarring.

EPIDEMIOLOGY AND ETIOLOGY
For the past 20 years, the proportion of patients with primary FSGS has risen from <10% to approximately 25% of adult nephropathies. FSGS is the most common form of idiopathic nephrotic syndrome in African-Americans.

PATHOGENESIS
FSGS may be either idiopathic or secondary to a number of different causes (e.g. heroin abuse, HIV infection, sickle cell disease, obesity, reflux of urine from the bladder to the kidneys, and lesions associated with single or remnant kidneys). As renal function declines, repeat biopsy specimens show more glomeruli with segmental sclerosing lesions and increased numbers of globally sclerotic glomeruli. By immuno-fluorescence staining, IgM and C3 are commonly trapped in the areas of glomerular sclerosis.

CLINICAL HISTORY
Patients present with either asymptomatic proteinuria or edema. The nephrotic syndrome occurs in about two-thirds of patients at presentation, hypertension in 30–50%, and micro-scopic hematuria in about 50%; GFR is decreased at presentation in 20–30% of patients. Complement levels and other serologic test results are normal.

PHYSICAL EXAMINATION
In secondary FSGS clinical features of the underlying disease may be obvious. As a consequence of the renal disease, edema, hypertension, signs of volume overload and/or uremia may be present.

DIFFERENTIAL DIAGNOSIS
The differential diagnosis includes minimal change disease, membranous nephropathy, amyloidosis, diabetic nephropathy, postinfectious glomerulonephritis, IgA nephropathy, and membranoproliferative glomerulonephritis.

INVESTIGATIONS
Consequences of the nephrotic syndrome are hypoalbuminemia, reduced immunoglobulin levels, and hypercholesterolemia. Serum complement components are generally normal; circulating immune complexes have been detected. Serologic testing for HIV infection should be obtained.

HISTOLOGY
This is characterized by the presence of glomerular lesions of focal distribution affecting only some of the glomeruli. The lesions predominate in the deeper cortex mainly affecting the juxtamedullary glomeruli. The most common pattern is for sclerosis in the perihilar regions (35). The glomerular tip lesion variant, consolidation confined to the segment adjacent to the origin of the proximal tubule, may have a more benign prognosis. Another variant, collapsing glomerulopathy, has segmental collapse of capillaries with hypertrophy and hyperplasia of overlying epithelial cells. Collapsing glomerulopathy may be idiopathic or associated with HIV infection, SLE, hepatitis C, and pamidronate therapy.

PROGNOSIS
A minority of patients experience a spontaneous remission of proteinuria, and eventually most untreated patients develop end-stage renal disease (ESRD) in 5–20 years from presentation. The degree of proteinuria is a predictor for the long-term clinical outcome. Patients with non-nephrotic range proteinuria have a more favorable course with renal survival of over 80% after 10 years of follow-up, whereas the majority of patients excreting >10 g of protein per day will reach end-stage renal disease within 3 years.

One of the most useful prognostic indicators for patients with FSGS is whether or not they attain a remission of their nephrotic syndrome (in one study <15% of patients who had complete or partial remission progressed to ESRD within 5 years; up to 50% who did not attain remission progressed to ESRD within 6 years). An elevated entry serum creatinine is associated with a poor long-term renal survival; serum creatinine concentration >1.3 mg/dl (114.9 μmol/l) have a lower renal survival rate than those with better renal function, regardless of the level of proteinuria (10-year renal survival rate of 27%

versus 100%). Using multivariate analysis, the entry level creatinine concentration may be a better predictor. The renal prognosis for collapsing glomerulopathy is particularly poor.

MANAGEMENT

The first step is to distinguish between primary and secondary FSGS. Patients with secondary FSGS have a hyperfiltration injury and should be treated with ACE inhibitors or angiotensin II receptor antagonists. The management of primary FSGS remains difficult. There is recent enthusiasm for the use of high-dose, prolonged corticosteroid therapy. Studies in which 6–12 month courses of corticosteroids and cytotoxics have been used have achieved up to a 40–60% remission rate of the nephrotic syndrome with preservation of long-term renal function. Alternatively, a trial of cyclosporine (cyclosporin)/tacrolimus may be considered for patients with heavy proteinuria but preserved renal function. ACE inhibitors may also provide a substantial reduction in proteinuria and a potential long-term benefit that may be equal to or greater than that of the immunosuppressive therapy. During relapses supportive treatment of the nephrotic syndrome must be given – diuretics, antihypertensives, anticoagulation, and lipid-lowering agents may be necessary.

There is a 20–30% risk of recurrent disease following renal transplantation. In patients with recurrent FSGS following transplantation, the use of plasma exchange has been successful in reducing proteinuria, although proteinuria tends to recur following discontinuation of the treatment. The best results have been obtained when plasma exchange is initiated as soon as proteinuria recurs. The role of plasma exchange in the treatment of patients with primary FSGS is unclear.

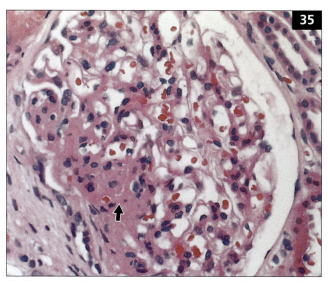

35 Glomerulus showing segmental sclerosis at the hilum (arrow). The remaining capillary tuft is normal. Light microscopy (H+E ×400).

Thin basement membrane nephropathy

DEFINITION
Thin glomerular basement membrane (GBM) disease, or thin membrane nephropathy, is characterized by isolated glomerular hematuria associated with a renal biopsy finding of excessively thin GBM.

EPIDEMIOLOGY AND ETIOLOGY
The condition is relatively common, with some authors estimating that thin GBM disease accounts for approximately 20–25% of patients evaluated for persistent isolated hematuria. It can present sporadically, or as a familial trait. When several members of the same family are affected, the condition is termed 'benign familial hematuria' (BFH). In patients with BFH, transmission follows an autosomal dominant pattern.

PATHOGENESIS
The pathogenesis is unclear. As opposed to patients with Alport's syndrome, immuno-histochemistry studies of type IV collagen in GBM of patients with thin GBM disease or with BFH have shown no abnormalities in the distribution of any of the six chains.

CLINICAL HISTORY
Clinical presentation is with persistent hematuria, first detected in childhood. In some cases, hematuria is intermittent and may not be manifested until adulthood. Macroscopic hematuria is not uncommon and may occur in association with an upper respiratory tract infection. When first detected in young adults, 60% have a level of proteinuria <500 mg/day.

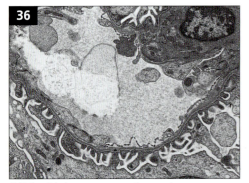

36 The thin basement membrane shows attenuation down to 120 nm, but preservation of the lamina rara externa and interna and the lamina densa. Electron microscopy (× 5000).

DIFFERENTIAL DIAGNOSIS
In sporadic cases, the differential diagnosis is with other causes of isolated hematuria, mainly IgA nephropathy. The main differential diagnosis of BFH is with Alport's syndrome. BFH is usually inherited as an autosomal dominant disorder with both genders equally affected. In patients with Alport's syndrome, electron microscopic studies can demonstrate progressive thickening and multilamellation of the GBM. Early on in the disease course, however, renal biopsy in patients with Alport's syndrome may show diffuse attenuation of the GBM, making the differential diagnosis difficult.

INVESTIGATION
The diagnosis of thin GBM disease can only be made by electron microscopic examination of a renal biopsy.

HISTOLOGY
Glomeruli appear normal on light and immuno-fluorescence microscopy. On electron microscopy, there is diffuse thinning of the lamina densa and of the GBM as a whole (**36**). It is important to recognize that GBM width varies with age and gender. The thickness of the lamina densa and of the GBM increases rapidly from birth until age 2 years, and then gradually into adulthood. In general, values of 373 ± 42 nm and 326 ± 45 nm are accepted as normal GBM thickness in adult males and females respectively. Reported data shows that patients with thin GBM nephropathy have a mean GBM thickness of 191 ± 28 nm. The decrease in GBM thickness is invariably due to a decrease of the lamina densa. Based on the above data, a GBM thickness ≤250 nm in an adult patient is considered strongly suggestive of thin GBM disease. In children, GBM thickness ranges from 200–250 nm.

PROGNOSIS
The vast majority of patients exhibit an excellent prognosis with renal function preserved long term. A very small minority of patients, however, exhibit progressive renal insufficiency, probably due to coincidental renal disease.

MANAGEMENT
Percutaneous renal biopsy is the definitive way to establish the diagnosis, but is not generally justified as these patients will usually have normal renal function. There is no specific treatment.

Membranous nephropathy

DEFINITION

Membranous nephropathy is a common immune-mediated glomerular disease and one of the leading causes of primary glomerular disease causing nephrotic syndrome in adults. It is a histologic diagnosis based on the presence of subepithelial deposits along the glomerular basement membrane.

EPIDEMIOLOGY AND ETIOLOGY

Membranous nephropathy is found in subjects of all ages, but it is most often diagnosed in middle-age with the peak incidence during the fourth and fifth decades of life, followed closely by the third and sixth decades. There is a 2:1 predominance of males to females diagnosed with the disease. Idiopathic membranous nephropathy affects all races.

PATHOGENESIS

Membranous nephropathy must be diagnosed by renal biopsy and is characterized by immune complex localization in the subepithelial zone of glomerular capillaries. The pathogenic mechanisms that cause this immune complex localization and the subsequent development of proteinuria and the nephrotic syndrome are not completely understood. The nature of the antigen involved in the immune complex deposits of membranous nephropathy and its source remain unknown. In fact, many different antigen–antibody combinations are likely to cause membranous nephropathy.

CLINICAL HISTORY

At presentation, proteinuria >2.0 g/day is found in 80–90% of patients at presentation, with >10 g found in as many as 30%. While over 90% of patients have no evidence of impaired renal function at the time of presentation, hypertension at onset is found in 13–55% of patients. A minority will have microscopic hematuria.

PHYSICAL EXAMINATION

Findings may vary from mild peripheral edema to full-blown nephrotic syndrome, including ascites, pericardial, and pleural effusions.

DIFFERENTIAL DIAGNOSIS

Membranous nephropathy occurs as an idiopathic (primary) or secondary disease. Secondary membranous glomerulopathy is caused by autoimmune diseases (e.g. systemic lupus erythematosus, autoimmune thyroiditis), infection (e.g. hepatitis B and C), drugs (e.g. penicillamine, gold, nonsteroidal anti-inflammatory drugs), and malignancies (e.g. colon cancer, lung cancer). In patients over the age of 60 years, membranous nephropathy is associated with a malignancy in 7–15% of patients.

INVESTIGATIONS

Similarly to other patients with nephrotic syndrome, hyperlipidemia is common. Renal impairment may be present. Lowered serum complement levels may suggest a diagnosis of SLE. Hepatitis B and C serology should be performed.

HISTOLOGY

Very early on in the disease process the glomeruli may be normal on light microscopy, and the diagnosis can be made only by immunofluorescence or electron microscopy. With more advanced lesions, capillary walls are thickened but capillary lumina are patent. On methenamine silver stain, subepithelial projections ('spikes') are seen along the capillary walls (**37**). The spikes represent deposition of new basement membrane material along the deposits. Crescent formation is rare and may be seen in association with anti-GBM antibodies. Immunohistochemistry shows marked granular deposition of

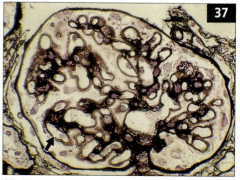

37 Glomerulus showing capillary wall thickening with well-developed subepithelial spike formation. Light microscopy (MS ×400).

Membranous nephropathy (*continued*)

IgG and C3 along the capillary walls (**38**). Electron microscopic features have been used to classify membranous nephropathy into four stages (**39–42**). In stage I, there are a few small-size subepithelial electron-dense deposits along the capillary walls, epithelial foot process effacement, but the glomeruli look normal on light microscopy. In stage II, deposits increase in number and size. There is formation of subepithelial projections of basement membrane by the side of the deposits ('spikes'). Stage III is characterized by extracellular material surrounding the deposits and incorporation of deposits into the capillary basement membrane. In stage IV, there is marked increase in capillary wall thickness, with the incorporated deposits becoming more lucent, and the spikes less apparent.

PROGNOSIS

Membranous nephropathy is considered a chronic disease, with the potential for spontaneous remission and relapsing episodes of the nephrotic syndrome. The renal prognosis is variable. In an analysis of 1,189 patients with membranous glomerulopathy pooled from across a number of clinical studies, the probability of renal survival was 86% at 5 years, 65% at 10 years and 59% at 15 years. It is likely, however, that the prognosis is even worse in nephrotic patients, since the risk of renal failure is correlated to the severity and the duration of proteinuria. Indeed, in approximately 15% of patients the disease has an accelerated course, with end-stage renal disease reached within one year from the diagnosis.

MANAGEMENT

Diuretics, antihypertensives, lipid lowering drugs, and anticoagulants are often used as a means of supportive care. When a secondary cause of MN is found, specific treatment of the underlying lesion may lead to remission of the nephropathy. The use of immunosuppression in the setting of idiopathic membranous glomerulopathy is controversial, especially because of the variable natural history of the disease and of drug toxicity. Immunosuppression is generally reserved for those patients with deteriorating renal function and/or heavy proteinuria. Various agents have been used including corticosteroids, cytotoxics such as cyclophosphamide, chlorambucil, and azathioprine or cyclosporine (cyclosporin).

The Italian Collaborative Study used alternating monthly courses of 1) methylprednisolone 1 g intravenously daily for 3 days, followed by oral prednisolone 0.5 mg/kg daily for the rest of the month, then 2) chlorambucil orally in a dose of 0.2 mg/kg daily for 1 month. This cycle was repeated until 6 months' treatment had been given. After 5 years follow-up, in the treated group (n=42), 14 were in remission, four had an increased creatinine >50% above baseline, with only one patient on dialysis. In the untreated group (n=39), four were in remission, 19 had an increased creatinine >50% above baseline, and four patients required dialysis. This is now a widely used if rather complicated regimen for MN. Recurrent disease is relatively rare following renal transplantation.

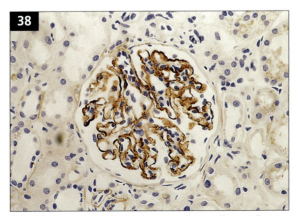

38 Global, granular IgG staining along the capillary walls (which is seen as a brown reaction product). Immunoperoxidase (anti-IgG antibody x400).

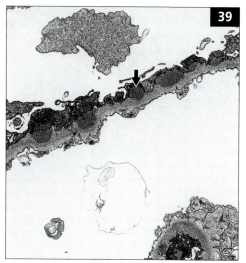

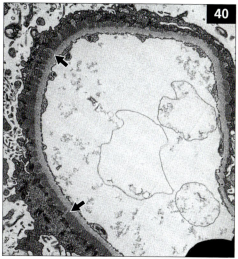

39 Stage I. Small electron-dense deposits are present along the subepithelial aspect of the capillary loop basement membrane (arrow). Visceral epithelial cell foot processes are diffusely effaced. Electron microscope appearance (×5800).

40 Stage II. Basement membrane 'spikes' separate the electron-dense deposits along the subepithelial aspect of the capillary loop basement membranes (arrows). Electron microscope appearance (×5800).

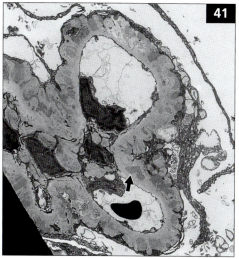

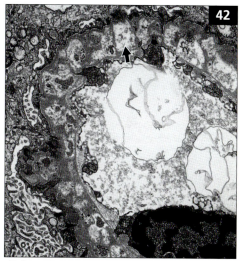

41 Stage III. Electron-dense deposits are completely incorporated within the thickened basement membrane (arrow). Electron microscope appearance (×3400).

42 Stage IV. Immune complex deposits are completely incorporated within the thickened capillary loop basement membranes. Most of the deposits have undergone reabsorption and are electron lucent (arrow). Electron microscope appearance (×7400).

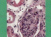

Membranoproliferative glomerulonephritis (MPGN)

DEFINITION
MPGN, also known as mesangiocapillary glomerulonephritis, is defined at the light microscopy level by the presence of diffuse mesangial proliferation and thickening of the glomerular capillary walls. MPGN may be primary (idiopathic) or secondary to specific diseases.

EPIDEMIOLOGY AND ETIOLOGY
The majority of patients with idiopathic type 1 MPGN are children between the ages of 8 and 16 years. It affects males and females equally. In the USA, Caucasians are relatively more affected than African-Americans. Secondary forms of type 1 MPGN tend to predominate in the adult population. The major cause of secondary MPGN is cryoglobulinemia due to HCV infection. Type 2 MPGN is a rare disease.

PATHOGENESIS
Type 1 MPGN appears to be an immune-mediated disease in which there is glomerular deposition of immune complexes in the mesangium and subendothelial space. Immune complex deposition results in complement activation with subsequent inflammation resulting in both proliferation of mesangial and endothelial cells and the recruitment of inflammatory cells, including neutrophils and monocytes. MPGN type 1 is most commonly associated with chronic immune-complex diseases like HCV, HBV, HIV, bacterial endocarditis, collagen vascular diseases, or malignancy. The pathogenesis of type 2 MPGN is linked to the chronic activation of the alternative pathway of complement. In most cases, there is a circulating autoantibody (C3 nephritic factors; C3Nef). This autoantibody binds to the alternative pathway C3 convertase preventing its inactivation, resulting in continuous complement activation and consumption. How this process results in the formation of characteristic 'dense deposits' in the GBM is unknown.

CLINICAL HISTORY
The clinical presentations of all forms of MPGN are variable and include nephrotic and nephritic features. Approximately one-third of the patients present with a combination of asymptomatic hematuria and proteinuria. Another third will present with nephrotic syndrome and preserved renal function. In about 20% of cases, patients will present with chronic renal failure. Some patients (~10%) will present with a nephritic syndrome picture, with hematuria, red blood cell casts,

hypertension, and renal insufficiency. An upper respiratory tract infection often precedes the first manifestation of the renal disease. Hypertension is common (50–80%). In patients with cryoglobulinemia and HCV infection, clinical manifestations resemble those of systemic vasculitis.

PHYSICAL EXAMINATION
Edema and hypertension are common. Patients with idiopathic MPGN type 2 may manifest partial lipodystrophy, usually limited to the face (**19**) and upper body. In secondary forms there may be signs of an associated neoplasm, hereditary disease, autoimmune disease, or infection. In patients with cryoglobulinemia palpable purpura, arthritis, hepatomegaly, digital necrosis, or vasculitic lesions may be present.

DIFFERENTIAL DIAGNOSIS
A number of pathologic conditions may cause an MPGN pattern on renal biopsy. The most important are poststreptococcal glomerulonephritis, thrombotic microangiopathies, paraproteinemias, SLE, mixed cryoglobulinemia, endocarditis, and chronic liver disease. Immunofluorescence and electron microscopy studies together with serology and clinical history should allow the correct diagnosis to be made. The diagnosis of MPGN should prompt a search for underlying bacterial or viral infections, especially HCV, HBV, and HIV. The absence of CH50 suggests an hereditary deficiency in one of the components of the complement cascade. Low complement levels can also be found in postinfectious glomerulonephritis, SLE, and following renal cholesterol emboli.

INVESTIGATIONS
In MPGN type 1, and in cryoglobulinemic MPGN, there are low C3, C4, and CH50 levels reflecting activation of both complement pathways. In MPGN type 2 the alternative pathway is activated, with patients having a persistently low C3 but normal C4 levels.

HISTOLOGY
Type 1 is the most common (**43**). There is diffuse global capillary wall thickening as a result of infiltrating leukocytes and intrinsic glomerular cell proliferation, leading to a lobular appearance of the glomeruli. The proliferating mesangial cells interpose their cell processes between the glomerular basement membrane and the endothelium ('mesangial interposition'), usually in association

with subendothelial deposits. The production of neomembrane by the endothelial cells results in a double contour or 'tram track' aspect, best seen on silver stain. Infiltrating mononuclear leukocytes and neutrophils also contribute to the glomerular hypercellularity. By immunofluorescence, there is granular deposition of IgG and C3 in the mesangium and outlining the lobular contours. IgM, IgA, C4 and C1q may also be found, but the staining is weaker and more variable. By electron microscopy, discrete immune deposits can be seen in the subendothelial space and in the mesangium (**44**).

Type 2 MPGN, also known as 'dense deposit disease', is characterized by the presence on electron microscopy of highly electron-dense deposits which replace the lamina densa and produce a smooth, ribbon-like thickening (**45**). Immunofluorescence shows intense capillary wall linear to band-like staining for C3, with little or no staining for C4 or immunoglobulins.

Type 3 MPGN is histologically similar to type 1 MPGN except that, in addition to the subendothelial space, deposits can also be seen within the glomerular basement membrane, and in the subepithelial space.

PROGNOSIS
MPGN type 1 tends to run a slowly progressive course with 40–50% of patients reaching ESRD in 10 years. Non-nephrotic patients have a better prognosis with 85% renal survival rate at 10 years. In adults the prognosis is less favorable, with near 50% of the patients reaching ESRD 5 years from diagnosis. Patients with MPGN type 2 have the worst prognosis. In these patients clinical remission rates are <5%. Predictors of poor outcome include impaired renal function at presentation, nephrotic range proteinuria, hypertension, number of crescents (>50%), and tubulointerstitial damage. MPGN type 1 frequently recurs after transplantation, resulting in loss of the allograft in over one-third of the patients. Recurrence is even more common in MPGN type 2 (80–100%), but allograft losses are less common.

MANAGEMENT
In children with idiopathic MPGN type 1, prolonged use of corticosteroids (up to 4 years) may lead to partial or complete clinical remission and stabilization of renal function. In adults, there is less convincing evidence for a role for corticosteroid therapy. The use of aspirin and dipyridamole is controversial. No therapy has been shown to be efficacious in type 2 or type 3 MPGN. In secondary forms of MPGN, treatment is dependent on the underlying condition.

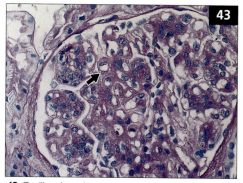

43 Capillary loop lumens are compromised due to endocapillary proliferation, leukocyte infiltration and basement membrane thickening with double-contouring (arrow). There is a generalized increase in mesangial cells and matrix. Light microscopy (PAS ×400).

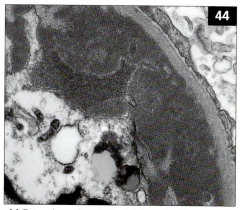

44 Extensive subendothelial deposits. Electron microscopy (×12,000).

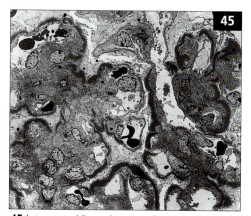

45 Interrupted linear, intramembranous electron-dense deposits. Electron microscopy (×1000).

Poststreptococcal glomerulonephritis (PSGN)

DEFINITION
Poststreptococcal glomerulonephritis is an acute glomerulonephritis that develops secondary to a pharyngitis or skin infection with specific strains of group A β-hemolytic streptococci. More recently, it has been shown that acute glomerulonephritis also occurs with non-group A streptococcus, particularly group C.

EPIDEMIOLOGY AND ETIOLOGY
While in developed countries the incidence of PSGN has decreased, it continues to be a significant public health problem in highly-populated areas with low socioeconomic status and poor sanitary conditions, particularly in the tropics. The disease is more common in children between age 5 and 15 years, but it can occur in all age groups. Unlike rheumatic fever, which can occur following a pharyngeal infection by any group A streptococci, PSGN occurs only with certain 'nephritogenic' strains of group A β-hemolytic streptococci (M type 1, 3, 4, 12, 25, and 49 in pharyngitis and 2, 49, 55, 57, and 60 with erysipelas and impetigo).

PATHOGENESIS
The specific pathogenic process responsible for the development of PSGN is unknown. Immune complex deposition, as well as autoimmune reactivity, is thought to play an important role in the disease process. Circulating IgG and C3 immune complexes have been demonstrated in patients with PSGN, but also in patients with documented streptococcal infection without renal compromise. It remains to be determined whether circulating immune complexes have an increased affinity for the glomerulus or whether streptococcal antigens can trigger the production of antibodies, which cross-react against glomerular antigens. It is also possible that streptococcal antigens may bind directly to glomerular sites forming *in situ* immune complexes that trigger an inflammatory response.

CLINICAL HISTORY
Onset is abrupt and is preceded by a streptococcus infection by approximately 1–4 weeks. The typical presentation is with a nephritic syndrome manifested by the presence of hematuria, oliguria, hypertension, edema, proteinuria, and azotemia. Oliguria is a frequent finding, but anuria is uncommon and, if persistent, suggests a rapidly progressive glomerulonephritis. The expanded extracellular fluid volume may cause cough, dyspnea, and orthopnea. Children may also develop fever, nausea, vomiting, abdominal pain, headache, encephalopathy, or seizures.

PHYSICAL EXAMINATION
The edema is typically periorbital and is worse in the morning. Weight gain may occur secondary to fluid retention. Hypertension is usually mild to moderate and is likely to be attributable to increased sodium and water retention. If fluid retention is severe, pleural effusions and pulmonary edema may develop.

DIFFERENTIAL DIAGNOSIS
Although traditionally the diagnosis of a diffuse proliferative endocapillary GN has been associated with streptococcal infection, similar histopathology occurs secondary to a number of other infective agents (*Table 4*). The differential diagnosis should also include other causes of nephritic syndrome such as IgA, Henoch–Schönlein purpura, idiopathic MPGN, and systemic vasculitis.

INVESTIGATIONS
Hematuria is present is almost all cases and may be macroscopic. Dysmorphic red cells (*7*), red cell casts (*8*), and white cell casts are common. Non-nephrotic proteinuria is common but it may be in the nephrotic range in some cases. Normocytic normochromic anemia is usually dilutional but may reflect shortening of the red blood cells' life-span secondary to rapid elimination of immune complex-coated cells. Cultures are usually negative but antibody titer to streptolysin O (ASO), anti-streptokinase, anti-

Table 4 Causes of postinfectious glomerulonephritis

Bacteria	Viruses
Streptococcus	Herpes zoster
Pneumococcus	Mumps
Staphylococcus	Hepatitis B
Klebsiella	Epstein–Barr
Brucella	Echovirus
Treponema	Coxsackie B4
Leptospira	Influenza
Salmonella	Cytomegalovirus
Mycoplasma	
Meningococcus	**Parasites**
Mycobacteria	Plasmodium falciparum
Gonococcus	Toxoplasma
	Echinococcus

hyaluronidase, anti-deoxyribonuclease, and anti-nicotyladenine dinucleotidase may provide evidence of recent streptococcal infection. ASO titers rise 10–14 days after infection and peak at 3–4 weeks with subsequent fall. Total hemolytic (CH50) complement and C3 levels are usually reduced, but C4 levels are normal.

HISTOLOGY

This is the classic example of an acute endocapillary proliferative glomerulonephritis. Light microscopy shows diffuse hypercellularity of the glomerular tufts, with mesangial and endothelial cell proliferation and infiltration of polymorphonuclear leukocytes (thus the name exudative), monocytes/macrophages, and plasma cells (**46**). All glomeruli are affected in a homogeneous pattern. Early on in the disease process, characteristic subepithelial 'humps' can be detected on silver stain. Cellular crescents are uncommon and their presence is indicative of severe disease. On immunohistochemistry, there is granular deposition of IgG, C3, and occasionally IgM, distributed in three well-described patterns: 'starry-sky', 'mesangial', and 'garland' (**47**). By electron microscopy, small immune deposits are seen in the mesangial and subendothelial areas. Almost pathognomonic of PSGN is the presence of large 'humps', which are dome-shape subepithelial deposits in the glomerular basement membrane (**48**).

PROGNOSIS

In children the prognosis is excellent with most patients recovering renal function within 1–2 months of diagnosis. In a few patients, especially adults, microscopic hematuria, proteinuria, hypertension, and renal dysfunction may persist for many years. Patients presenting with a crescentic nephritis have a poorer prognosis, with approximately 50% developing ESRD. In contrast with rheumatic fever, where the risk of recurrence is life-long, PSGN does not recur following subsequent streptococcal infections.

MANAGEMENT

The treatment of PSGN is supportive. Appropriate antibiotic therapy is indicated if there is persistent infection. Sodium restriction and the use of loop diuretics reduce the risk of fluid overload and help to control hypertension. Renal function is impaired, but only 5% of the patients will require dialysis to control hyperkalemia or fluid overload. The presence of crescents is an ominous sign. In a few case reports, the use of corticosteroids, cyclophosphamide, and plasmapheresis improved prognosis in patients with a crescentic glomerulonephritis.

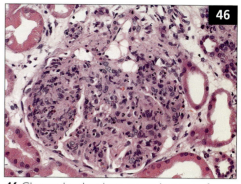

46 Glomerulus showing a severe increase of cellularity with numerous infiltrating polymorphs. Light microscopy (H+E ×400).

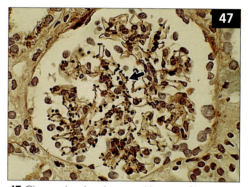

47 Glomerulus showing round humps of brown reaction product on the epithelial side of capillary walls (arrow). Immunoperoxidase (anti-IgG antibody ×350).

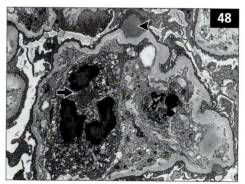

48 Glomerular capillary tuft containing a polymorph (arrow) and showing a subepithelial hump (arrow head). Electron microscopy (×4000).

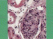

IgA nephropathy

DEFINITION
IgA nephropathy (IgAN), or Berger's disease, is defined as a mesangial proliferative glomerulonephritis characterized by diffuse deposition of IgA in the mesangium.

EPIDEMIOLOGY AND ETIOLOGY
It is the most common primary glomerular disease worldwide and accounts for approximately 10% of patients reaching ESRD in many countries. The general prevalence may be as high as 1:100 people. It occurs in all age groups, but is most commonly diagnosed in patients in their second or third decades of life (80% 16–35 years old). Males are more frequently affected. There is wide geographic variation. It is the most common primary glomerular diseases in Asia (30–40% cases), followed by Europe (20%), and North America (10%). IgAN is rare in central Africa and in African-Americans. A familial form has been described.

PATHOGENESIS
The pathogenesis of IgAN is poorly understood but a pivotal role is played by IgA. Increase in IgA1 concentration in the serum, increase in IgA1-containing circulating immune complexes and positive IgA–rheumatoid factor have all been described in patients with IgAN. In patients with IgAN, a number of studies have demonstrated abnormalities in the hinge region of the IgA1 molecule. This region (not present in IgA2) is composed of 18 amino acids of which five are serine or threonine glycosylation sites, O-linked to N-acetylgalactosamine (GalNAc). The oligosaccharide chain is usually extended by addition of a variable number of galactose (Gal) molecules and sialic acid residues to GalNAc, resulting in several hinge region glycoforms. Both deficiency in sialic acid with normal Gal content, or diminished Gal content in the IgA1 hinge region, have been reported in patients with IgAN. Recently it has been shown that mesangial IgA1 in IgAN exhibits aberrant O-glycosylation. The mechanism responsible for the abnormal glycosylation is unclear. A decrease in the activity of $\beta 1,3$ galactosyltransferase in B-cells obtained from patients with IgAN has been reported.

There are a number of potential reasons why abnormalities in O-glycosylation may be pathogenic in IgAN. Hypogalactosylation of IgA reduces the physiologic clearance of IgA1 molecules by the hepatocyte asialoglycoprotein receptor, thus resulting in an increase in circulating IgA. Decreased IgA1 glycosylation increases the tendency of IgA1 to aggregate and form macromolecules of IgA1 complexes. In addition, IgG antiglycan antibodies interact with hinge regions deficient in Gal and sialic acid forming IgA–IgG immune complexes. The mechanism by which IgA1 deposits in the glomeruli is unclear. Specific mesangial IgA1 receptors that recognize hinge region glycans have been described. Changes in the carbohydrate structure of immunoglobulins are known to modify interactions with cell surface receptors. Underglycosylation and desialylation of the IgA1 hinge region increases the propensity for binding to extracellular matrix components, and promotes glomerular deposition. Once the aberrant IgA1 is deposited in the glomeruli, it triggers traditional mediators of inflammation. Deposition of C3 and properdin without C4 suggests alternative complement pathway activation. Interleukin-1, interleukin-6, platelet-derived growth factor, tumor necrosis factor, free oxygen radicals, vascular cell adhesion molecule-1, and membrane attack complex (C5b-9) are a few of the factors implicated as modulators of the disease activity.

CLINICAL HISTORY
The classical presentation is episodic macroscopic hematuria, usually accompanying an intercurrent upper respiratory tract infection. This typical clinical pattern occurs most frequently in young adults in their second and third decades of life. Other patients are asymptomatic and may be identified when microscopic hematuria with or without proteinuria are found on a routine urinalysis. Proteinuria is common but nephrotic syndrome occurs in <10% of all cases. Patients may present with chronic renal failure.

DIFFERENTIAL DIAGNOSIS
Mesangial IgA occurs in other conditions, particularly in a number of autoimmune and inflammatory diseases, possibly as a result of increased IgA production or decreased clearance of circulating IgA. The most common causes of secondary IgAN are: gastrointestinal diseases (alcoholic cirrhosis, inflammatory bowel diseases, celiac disease), rheumatoid diseases (Reiter's, ankylosing spondylitis, psoriasis), malignancies (carcinomas, monoclonal IgA gammopathy), dermatitis herpetiformis, pulmonary hemosiderosis, mycosis fungoides, and infections

(HIV, hepatitis B, schistosomiasis). Other conditions that clinically can simulate IgAN include thin basement membrane disease and some forms of hereditary nephritis (e.g. Alport's).

INVESTIGATIONS

There are no specific laboratory findings for IgAN. Urinalysis shows persistent hematuria and dysmorphic red blood cells, associated with some degree of proteinuria. Serum IgA levels are increased in up to 50% of patients, but it is not specific. Serum complement levels are normal.

HISTOLOGY

Light microscopy findings are variable. The glomeruli may look normal or may show mesangial expansion secondary to mesangial cells proliferation, increased mesangial matrix, or both (**49**). The abnormalities may be global or segmental. Segmental sclerosing lesions are common. Tubulointerstitial findings correlate with the degree of glomerular damage. Occasionally, there is proliferation of the glomerular epithelial cells with crescent formation, but circumferential crescents are rare. Acute tubular necrosis has been documented in patients developing acute renal failure during an episode of heavy glomerular hematuria from crescentic IgAN. The diagnosis of IgAN requires immunohistochemistry showing IgA as the predominant or sole immunoglobulin deposit in the glomerular mesangium (**50**). In most cases, a second immunoglobulin (IgG or IgM) is also detected. Staining for C3 frequently, but not always, coincides with the IgA deposits. Staining for C1q is rare and helps to distinguish IgAN from lupus nephritis. On electron microscopy, electron-dense deposits in the mesangial and paramesangial areas co-localize with the immune deposits (**51**). In some cases, there is focal thinning, splitting, and lamination of the glomerular basement membrane.

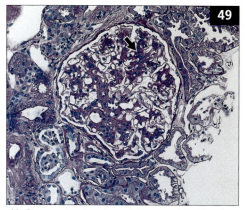

49 Glomerulus showing mild mesangial cell and matrix expansion (arrow). Light microscopy (PAS ×200).

50 Glomerulus showing IgA deposition in mesangial areas. Immunoperoxidase (anti-IgA antibody ×350).

51 Electron-dense deposits are identified within mesangial regions (arrow). Electron microscopy (×5800).

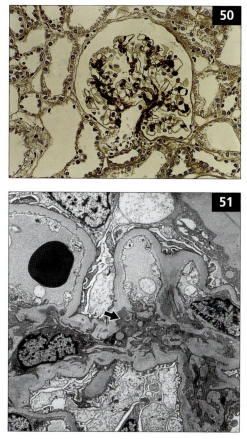

IgA nephropathy (*continued*)

PROGNOSIS

Actuarial curves of renal survival suggest 5–15% of patients with ESRD after 5 years from the apparent onset of the disease, 10–20% after 10 years, 15–30% after 15 years, and 20–50% after 20 years. Of the clinical and laboratory features included in multivariate analyses, baseline 24-hour proteinuria exceeding 1 g, hypertension, impaired renal function at diagnosis, and glomerular or interstitial fibrosis on renal biopsy, are the most important predictors of a poor outcome. IgAN recurs in about 50% of patients following renal transplantation but early loss of the allograft from recurrent disease is uncommon.

MANAGEMENT

Standard treatment includes treatment of hypertension, use of ACE inhibitors and angiotensin II receptor antagonists, and treatment of hyperlipidemia. Other treatments remain controversial. In a recent trial, 6 months of alternate-day corticosteroids in patients at risk of progression was beneficial in protecting renal function. In some series, treatment with fish oil has also been shown to be effective in providing long-term renal protection to patients with proteinuria and rising serum creatinine. Cyclosporine (cyclosporin) reduces proteinuria but its effect is likely to be hemodynamic secondary to reduction in GFR. Mycophenolate mofetil is currently undergoing clinical trials in patients with IgAN. Patients with IgAN and concomitant minimal-change disease respond fully to corticosteroids therapy. For patients with rapidly progressive renal failure due to crescentic IgAN, cortiosteroids and cyclophosphamide with the addition of plasma exchange or pulse methylprednisolone has been tried, with variable results.

Chapter Three

Systemic diseases affecting the glomeruli

- **Diabetes mellitus**

- **Plasma cell dyscrasias**

- **Amyloidosis**

- **Fibrillary and immunotactoid glomerulopathy**

- **Systemic lupus erythematosus (SLE)**

- **Primary anti-phospholipid antibody syndrome (PAPS)**

- **Systemic vasculitis**

- **Sickle cell anemia and glomerulonephritis**

- **Goodpasture's disease**

- **Glomerulonephritis associated with hepatitis B virus infection**

- **Glomerulonephritis associated with hepatitis C virus infection**

- **Glomerulonephritis associated with human immunodeficiency virus (HIV)**

- **Miscellaneous infections and glomerulonephritis**

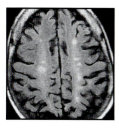
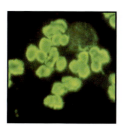
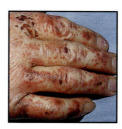
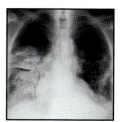

Diabetes mellitus

DEFINITION
Diabetic nephropathy is a common but not invariable complication of both type 1 and 2 diabetes mellitus. Clinically it presents with hypertension, proteinuria, edema and progressive renal impairment.

EPIDEMIOLOGY AND ETIOLOGY
Today diabetic nephropathy is the commonest cause of end-stage renal failure in the Western world. This is largely due to the epidemic of obesity and type 2 diabetes, and better survival of diabetics so that they reach end-stage renal failure. The epidemiology of diabetic nephropathy is easiest to study in type 1 diabetes, as the time of clinical onset is generally known. Between 25–45% of such patients will develop clinically evident disease as defined by overt proteinuria, and a further 20–30% will have subclinical microalbuminuria. The peak onset of nephropathy is between 10–15 years after the initial presentation with diabetes. Those individuals who do not have proteinuria at 25 years are very unlikely to develop nephropathy subsequently. The natural history is probably very similar in type 2 diabetics, although some groups have a worse prognosis. For example, nephropathy develops in 50% of Pima Indians at 20 years, with 15% having developed end-stage renal failure by this time. Risk factors for developing diabetic nephropathy include a positive family history of diabetic nephropathy, hypertension, poor glycemic control, and race (increased risk especially in blacks).

PATHOGENESIS
Hyperglycemia stimulates mesangial cell matrix production and also leads to increased glycosylation of proteins, leading to accumulation of advanced glyosylation end products which can cross-link with collagen. Another pathway by which hyperglycemia may trigger damage is the polyol pathway, leading to increased sorbitol concentrations. The initial physiologic abnormality is glomerular hyperfiltration due to an increase in renal volume and renal blood flow.

CLINICAL HISTORY
Type 1 diabetics normally are first noted to have microalbuminuria and subsequently proteinuria when they attend the diabetic clinic. The proteinuria can become nephrotic range, and the degree of proteinuria is roughly related to prognosis. Renal insufficency is generally progressive, but the rate of decline varies between individual patients. As renal failure develops typical uremic symptoms and signs develop, and diabetics seem to tolerate uremia worse than nondiabetics, developing symptoms at lower creatinine levels. Type 2 diabetics are often asymptomatic for many years before presenting to medical attention. Therefore, when they are first seen they may already have proteinuria or renal impairment.

Symptomatic urinary tract infections are more severe in diabetics and may be complicated by papillary necrosis, acute pyelonephritis, or perirenal abscess formation.

PHYSICAL EXAMINATION
Type 1 diabetics with nephropathy almost invariably have other signs of diabetic microvascular disease such as retinopathy (**52, 53**) and neuropathy. The relation of retinopathy to nephropathy is not so consistent in type 2 diabetes. Uremic polyneuropathy is often superimposed on the diabetic neuropathy. There is a 'glove and stocking' pattern of loss of sensation. Neuropathic foot lesions are due to lack of sensation causing recurrent trauma. Autonomic neuropathy is a common and troublesome problem affecting bowel, bladder, and sexual function.

The majority of patients with diabetic nephropathy will suffer from hypertension. Atherosclerosis is accelerated in uremic diabetics and there is a very high incidence of cerebrovascular, coronary, renovascular, and peripheral vascular disease.

DIFFERENTIAL DIAGNOSIS
Since diabetes mellitus is very common, it can co-exist with other renal diseases, especially in the elderly. In the presence of the appropriate clinical history and diabetic retinopathy, a renal biopsy is not usually needed. If a diabetic has coincident microscopic hematuria, and especially red cell casts, it is likely that they have concurrent nondiabetic renal disease such as IgA nephropathy. If renal size is asymmetric on renal ultrasound, renal arterial stenosis should be excluded.

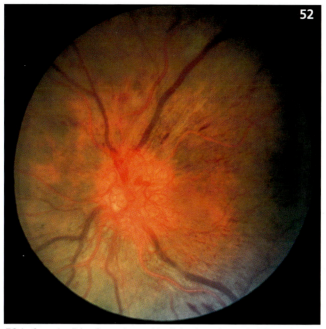

52 Left optic disk of a patient with diabetic retinopathy. There is gross neovascularization of the disc with retinal hemorrhages and cotton wool spots.

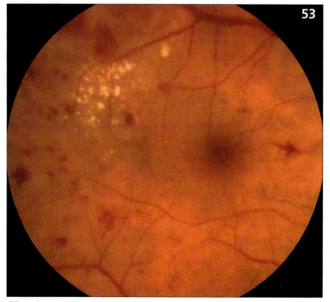

53 Left optic disc of another patient with diabetic retinopathy. There is extensive background retinopathy with hard exudation and hemorrhage temporal to the macula, indicating some retinal ischemia.

Diabetes mellitus (*continued*)

INVESTIGATIONS

Microalbuminuria is detected by a sensitive radioimmunoassay. Albumin excretion rate in normoalbuminuria is <20 µg/min, microalbuminuria 20–200 µg/min, and proteinuria >200 µg/min. If 24 hour urine collections are performed, albumin excretion rate in normoalbuminuria is <30 mg/24 h, micro-albuminuria 30–300 mg/24 h, and proteinuria >300 mg/24 h. There is a circadian rhythm and considerable day-to-day variation in albumin excretion. Therefore the diagnosis of microalbuminuria depends on finding increased rates of excretion in at least three collections over a 6-month period.

Renal function should be measured by creatinine clearance or GFR measurement. Urinalysis for microscopic hematuria and red cell casts and renal ultrasonography should be performed.

HISTOLOGY (54–57)

In the earliest stage of the disease there is glomerular hypertrophy and thickening of the glomerular basement membrane. As the disease progresses, these changes are followed by hyalinosis of the afferent and efferent arterioles. Later changes include exudative lesions which occur within the capillary loop as hyaline caps and on the surface of Bowman's capsule as capsular drops. There is progressive mesangial expansion causing diffuse diabetic glomerulosclerosis. Sometimes the mesangial expansion shows a nodular appearance; these are Kimmelstiel–Wilson nodules, which are pathognomonic of diabetic nephropathy, but only occur in a minority of biopsies. Both the diffuse and nodular mesangial expansion are composed of extra mesangial matrix, which stains positively with silver and PAS. Electron microscopy will show an increase in basement membrane thickness.

PROGNOSIS

Untreated patients with diabetic nephropathy will progress to end-stage renal failure. The rate of decline from developing fixed proteinuria to end-stage renal failure varies from months to decades, with a mean of about 5 years.

MANAGEMENT

Progression of diabetic nephropathy can be retarded by tight glycemic control, use of angiotensin-converting enzyme inhibitors or angiotensin receptor antagonists and good blood pressure control (target 130/80 mmHg [17.3/10.7 kPa]). Diabetics with end-stage renal failure can be managed either with hemodialysis or peritoneal dialysis. Patients who receive a combined kidney–pancreas transplant have been shown to have a survival advantage over diabetics who receive a kidney transplant, probably due to a reduction in cardiovascular events. Islet cell transplants are currently in an exciting phase of clinical development.

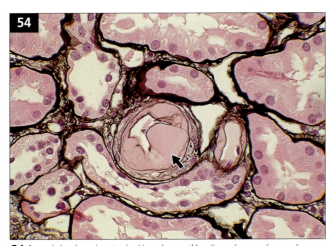

54 Arteriole showing typical 'exuberant' hyaline change (arrow). Light microscopy (MS ×400).

55 Glomerulus showing hyaline nodules in both afferent and efferent arterioles (arrows). Light microscopy (MS ×400).

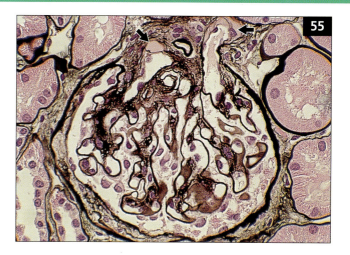

56 Glomerulus showing silver positive nodular lesions (arrow) (Kimmelstiel Wilson nodules). Light microscopy (MS ×400).

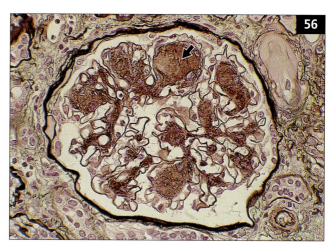

57 Glomerulus showing diffuse increase of mesangial matrix (diffuse diabetic glomerulosclerosis) and a capsular drop (PAS-positive exudative lesion) (arrow). Light microscopy (PAS ×400).

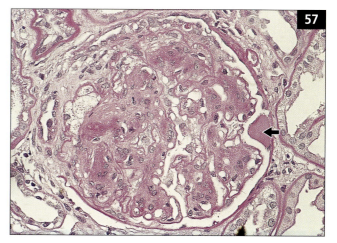

Plasma cell dyscrasias

DEFINITION

Plasma cell dyscrasias are diseases caused by clonal proliferation of plasma cells and their precursors, activated B-cells, which secrete unique immunoglobulin proteins or immunoglobulin light or heavy chains. Renal disease occurs commonly in multiple myeloma, primary amyloidosis, and light chain deposition disease. Primary amyloidosis will be discussed separately.

EPIDEMIOLOGY AND ETIOLOGY

Myeloma has an incidence of about 2–4/100,000 and is a disease of the elderly, reaching a peak incidence in the eighth decade in men. Immunophenotyping indicates that the myeloma cells are clones of B-cells that are late in their differentiation pathway. Chromosomal translocations affecting the immunoglobulin heavy chain locus on the long arm of chromosome 14 are found in 20–60% of patients; deletion of chromosome 13 or translocation of chromosome 1q are associated with worse outcome, as are mutations in ras, p53, or retinoblastoma tumor suppressor genes. It is thought that the abnormal B-cells originate in lymph nodes and migrate to the bone marrow which provides a cytokine-rich microenvironment that allows the cells to proliferate.

PATHOGENESIS

Myeloma can affect kidney function by several mechanisms. Myeloma kidney refers to the commonest type of renal injury in which large intratubular casts are formed. The tubular injury is caused by Bence Jones proteins. Cast nephropathy only develops in some patients. It is thought that the physicochemic properties of the proteins as well as host factors explain this.

Bence Jones proteinuria may rarely affect proximal tubular function to cause Fanconi syndrome. Hypercalcemia is common in myeloma due to secretion of osteoclast activating factor causing increased bone reabsorption. Hypercalcemia leads to polyuria and volume depletion, and also causes vasoconstriction in the renal circulation. Myeloma patients are particularly susceptible to radiographic contrast causing acute renal failure. Light chains may form nodular deposits in the glomeruli (light chain deposition disease), or be enzymatically degraded into amyloid proteins which polymerize into amyloid fibrils (AL amyloid).

CLINICAL HISTORY

Patients with myeloma classically present with skeletal pain or pathologic fractures. Hypogammaglobulinemia in these patients predisposes them to infections. Renal disease in myeloma can present as mild proteinuria with or without hematuria, nephrotic syndrome, slowly progressive renal insufficiency, or acute renal failure. Renal disease is present in 50% of patients at presentation. Most commonly renal insufficiency progresses insidiously; acute renal failure occurs in <10% of patients.

PHYSICAL EXAMINATION

Anemia is common, and there may be an enhanced bleeding tendency leading to spontaneous bruising.

DIFFERENTIAL DIAGNOSIS

The diagnosis of multiple myeloma is made by finding >10% plasma cells in the bone marrow, or a plasmacytoma together with one of the following: a monoclonal protein in the blood or urine, or lytic bone lesions. Connective tissue diseases, metastatic cancer, lymphoma, or leukemia may share some clinical features with myeloma. Multiple myeloma also needs to be distinguished from monoclonal gammopathy of uncertain significance, smouldering multiple myeloma, and primary amyloidosis.

INVESTIGATIONS

A standard myeloma workup includes a full blood count, serum creatinine and calcium, serum electrophoresis and paraprotein quantification, a 24-hour urine collection for electrophoresis and immunofixation, a bone marrow examination, and a skeletal survey (58). Light chains are typically not detected by urine dipsticks. They are precipitated by sulphosalicylic acid. Immunofixation is now the method of detection for light chains. In contrast, patients with primary amyloidosis will have increased albumin excretion detected by routine urinalysis.

HISTOLOGY

Myeloma cast nephropathy is characterized by large, eosinophilic refractile casts that frequently show fractures (so called 'hard' casts), which are found mainly in the distal convoluted tubules and collecting ducts (59). The casts often incite a 'foreign body' giant cell reaction, and there is usually a dense interstitial cellular infiltrate consisting of mononuclear cells and macro-

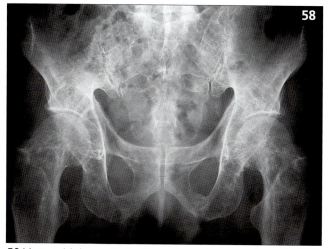

58 X-ray pelvis in a patient with myeloma demonstrating multiple lytic lesions.

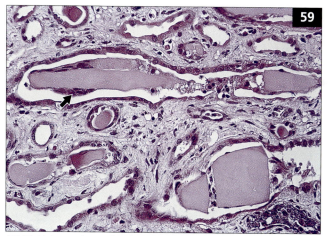

59 Multiple myeloma. Cortical tubules contain 'hard' eosinophilic casts which have fractured and incited a 'foreign body' giant cell reaction (arrow). Notice the tubular epithelial cell damage and the interstitial fibrosis. Light microscopy (H+E x350).

Plasma cell dyscrasias (*continued*)

phages. Proximal and distal tubular cells may be flattened with areas of necrosis and denudation of the tubular basement membrane.

Light chain deposition disease (**60–62**) is characterized by the finding on immuno-histochemistry of diffuse linear staining of the basement membranes of tubules, Bowman's capsule, and glomerular capillaries for a single light chain isotype. Nodular glomerulo-sclerosis, superficially resembling diabetic nephropathy on light microscopy, is only found in about 60% of patients. Silver staining frequently allows these to be distinguished because the nodules in diabetes are silver-positive and in light chain disease are negative. Electron microscopy will show granular electron-dense material on glomerular and tubular basement membranes.

PROGNOSIS
Adverse prognostic factors in multiple myeloma include the presence of plasma cells in the peripheral blood, renal failure, infection, and increased age. Treatment regimes include corticosteroids and melphalan, high-dose chemotherapy, and autologous bone marrow transplantation.

The prognosis for patients with light chain deposit disease depends on the severity of the renal lesion and degree of systemic involvement, with liver and heart failure common.

MANAGEMENT
Treatment aimed at improving renal function includes correction of hypovolemia, stopping nephrotoxic drugs, forced alkaline diuresis, and reduction of light chain levels by chemotherapy and plasmapheresis.

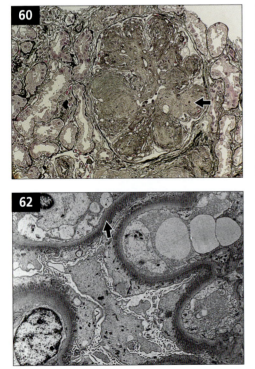

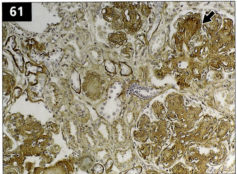

60 Glomerulus showing silver-negative nodules (arrow) (compare with diabetic nodules). Light microscopy (MS x400).

61 Glomeruli from the same patient as **60** showing positive staining (brown reaction product) of nodules and glomerular capillary walls (arrow). Light microscopy (Peroxidase/anti-kappa antibody x250).

62 Granular diffuse subendothelial electron-dense material (arrow). Electron microscopy (x4000).

Amyloidosis

DEFINITION

Amyloid consists of the deposition in the extracellular space of a waxy insoluble polymerized protein, the nature of which relates to the underlying etiology. Amyloid stains pink with hematoxylin–eosin and red with Congo red, which also shows a characteristic apple-green/orange birefringence when viewed with polarized light. Electron microscopy shows nonbranching fibrils. X-ray diffraction analysis shows that the fibrils have a beta-pleated sheet pattern. The amyloid material that accumulates in the extracellular compartment progressively destroys the involved organ, but interestingly does not incite an inflammatory reaction.

EPIDEMIOLOGY AND ETIOLOGY

Primary amyloidosis (AL) can occur in patients without overt, underlying disease or during the course of multiple myeloma. The underlying disease process is the clonal proliferation of plasma cells in both groups, since a serum paraprotein is found in 90% of patients in the group without myeloma. The median age at presentation is 65 years, and is more common in males.

Secondary amyloidosis (AA) complicates chronic inflammatory conditions such as rheumatoid arthritis, ankylosing spondylitis, bronchiectasis, osteomyelitis, paraplegia with chronic skin ulceration, malignancies such as Hodgkin's disease and renal cell carcinoma, and familial Mediterranean fever.

PATHOGENESIS

Amyloid fibrils are composed of specific proteins produced in certain disease states, a serum amyloid P protein (SAP) common to all systemic forms of amyloid, and small amounts of glycosaminoglycans.

For instance, in AL amyloid, which is associated with the production of an abnormal paraprotein, the amyloid is formed by the polymerizationof light chains or portions of light chain. In this instance the amyloid is unique to each patient.

In AA amyloid the polymerizing protein is identical in all patients and is serum amyloid A protein (SAA) that is produced in the liver (an acute phase reactant).

CLINICAL HISTORY AND PHYSICAL EXAMINATION

The most common presenting symptoms are weight loss and fatigue. Symptoms and signs of congestive cardiac failure, nephrotic syndrome, autonomic neuropathy, gastrointestinal involvement, peripheral neuropathy, or carpal tunnel syndrome may be present. Macroglossia occurs in about 10% of cases of AL amyloid. Hepatosplenomegaly may occur. Periorbital purpura is common.

Renal involvement usually presents with nephrotic syndrome, which persists despite progression to renal insufficiency. Renal vein thrombosis is a common complication.

DIFFERENTIAL DIAGNOSIS

Although amyloid is usually deposited in multiple organs it may present with single organ involvement, e.g. nephrotic syndrome. A careful history will usually reveal an underlying cause for AA amyloid. Tissue biopsy is necessary to reach a precise diagnosis, although SAP scanning (see below) may be an alternative when biopsy is not possible. Positive immunohistochemic staining of biopsy material using antibodies to AA protein confirms AA amyloid. Negative staining implies AL amyloid. This may be confirmed by demonstrating positive staining with either anti-kappa or lambda antibodies; however, this is frequently unsatisfactory.

INVESTIGATIONS

In AL amyloid immunoelectrophoresis and immunofixation of both serum and urine will detect a monoclonal protein in 90% of cases. A bone marrow aspiration should be done to determine whether a clonal plasma cell proliferation is present and to stain for amyloid. In the presence of renal involvement, a renal biopsy is normally performed. Ultrasound usually shows bilaterally enlarged kidneys. Less invasive sites that can be biopsied include abdominal fat pad or rectum which are both positive in 80% of patients. Serum CRP or SAA concentrations can be used to follow the activity of the underlying inflammatory process.

Radioiodinated SAP specifically localizes to amyloid deposits and can be used to measure

Amyloidosis (*continued*)

the total body amyloid burden (amount and organ distribution) and serial scans can be used to follow progression or regression with treatment (**63**). SAP is not effective for visualizing cardiac deposits and echocardiography is needed for this.

HISTOLOGY (64–67)
The principal site of renal involvement is quite variable. Generally amyloid first deposits in the glomerular mesangium and then extends out into the capillary loops when it is associated with a protein leak. At a later stage nodules may be formed. It is also found along the tubular basement membrane, when it may be associated with tubular atrophy, and in the walls of arterioles and venules. Electron microscopy reveals regular nonbranched fibrils measuring 7.5–10 nm in width and 30–1000 nm in length.

PROGNOSIS
The median survival for AL patients is about 2 years, with adverse prognostic factors including cardiac failure, renal impairment, hepatomegaly, and diagnosis of multiple myeloma. Most patients with renal involvement progress to end-stage renal failure rapidly.

MANAGEMENT
The goal of treatment in AL patients is to decrease the synthesis of the amyloidogenic light chain. Similar approaches are used in the treatment of myeloma and AL amyloid, with encouraging results with the use of autologous stem cell transplantation in selected patients.

In AA amyloid, therapy is aimed at controlling the underlying disease as this can lead to stabilizationor regression of the amyloidosis. Colchicine is used to treat familial Mediterranean fever. Renal transplantation has been performed in selected patients with AA amyloid, as recurrence of amyloidosis tends not to cause clinical problems until late after transplantation.

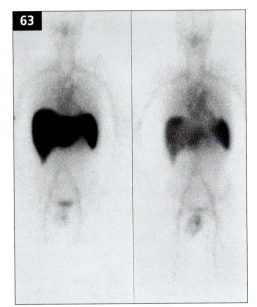

63 Serial anterior whole body I^{125}-serum amyloid P component scintigraphy demonstrating regression of hepatic and splenic AA amyloid deposits in a patient with rheumatoid arthritis. Inflammatory disease activity was completely suppressed by treatment with oral chlorambucil in 1998 and the follow-up scan on the right was performed 2 years later.

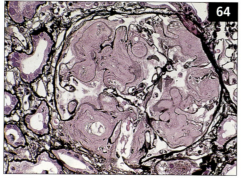

64 Glomerulus showing severe eosinophilic, silver-negative mesangial expansion and capillary wall thickening. Light microscopy (MS ×400).

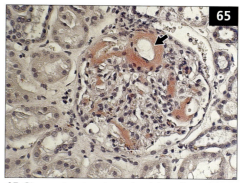

65 Glomerulus showing red staining of arteriole (arrow) and segmental staining of the mesangium. Light microscopy (Congo red ×350).

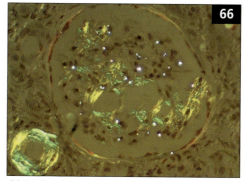

66 Similar glomerulus to **65** viewed by crossed polarized prisms showing characteristic green/yellow birefringence (Congo red ×350).

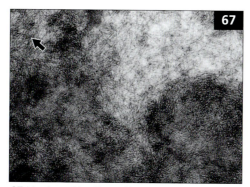

67 Nonbranching fibers 12 nm in diameter. Electron microscopy (×20,000).

Fibrillary and immunotactoid glomerulopathy

DEFINITION
Fibrillary glomerulonephritis is characterized by the appearance on electron microscopy in the mesangium of randomly arranged fibrils that are larger than those in amyloidosis (20–30 nm versus 10 nm in diameter) and do not stain with Congo red. Immunotactoid glomerulopathy is characterized by the formation of microtubules (30–40 nm in diameter).

EPIDEMIOLOGY AND ETIOLOGY
It is controversial whether fibrillary glomerulonephritis and immunotactoid glomerulopathy are separate disorders. Fibrillary glomerulonephritis accounts for 85% of cases. It occurs principally in adults. In one centre's biopsy series it occurred in 1% of biopsies.

PATHOGENESIS
Immunohistochemistry in cases of fibrillary glomerulonephritis is characterized by IgG4 subclass deposition, suggesting this may be key in fibril formation. Patients with immunotactoid glomerulopathy may have either a circulating paraprotein or monoclonal immunoglobulin deposition, and there is a disease association with B-cell lymphoma or chronic lymphocytic leukemia.

CLINICAL HISTORY
Patients with these conditions may present with proteinuria usually with associated microscopic hematuria, hypertension, or progressive renal insufficiency. About 50% of patients develop end-stage renal failure within 2 years.

HISTOLOGY
The light microscopic appearances are variable and include: mesangial hypercellularity, amorphous, eosinophilic, Congo red-negative expansion of the mesangium, sometimes showing a nodular pattern, mesangiocapillary pattern, or crescent formation. Immunohistochemistry in cases of fibrillary glomerulonephropathy may be positive for IgG, C3, and light chains. Electron microscopy (**68**) is required for definitive diagnosis and shows a fibrillar pattern, similar to amyloid, but usually the fibrils have a greater diameter, perhaps up to 20 nm.

PROGNOSIS
About 50% of patients develop end-stage renal failure within 2 years.

MANAGEMENT
There is no proven effective treatment. Although recurrent disease in the renal allograft is common, the rate of progression is slow, and transplantation has been successful.

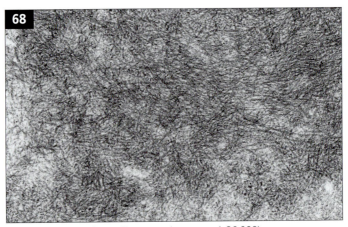

68 Nonbranching fibers. Electron microscopy (×20,000).

Systemic lupus erythematosus (SLE)

DEFINITION

Systemic lupus erythematosus is an autoimmune disease characterized by autoantibody production in which renal involvement is common. According to the American Rheumatism Association classification, a diagnosis of SLE is made if four of the following 11 criteria are present:

- Malar rash.
- Discoid rash.
- Photosensitivity.
- Oral ulcers.
- Arthritis (two or more joints).
- Pleurisy–pericarditis.
- Renal abnormalities.
- Neurologic disorders (seizures, psychosis).
- Hematologic disorders (hemolytic anemia, leucopenia, lymphocytopenia, thrombocytopenia).
- Immunologic disorders (anti-DNA, anti-Sm, positive finding of anti-phospholipid antibodies).
- Anti-nuclear antibody.

EPIDEMIOLOGY AND ETIOLOGY

SLE is about nine times more common in females than in males. The deleterious effect of estrogens on SLE explains the flares of disease activity with pregnancy or the use of oral contraception. All ages are affected but most cases occur between ages 16 and 55 years. There is a much higher incidence in black and Asian populations compared to Caucasians in the UK. There are certain HLA associations and some familial cases are associated with defects of the complement pathway. Exposure to sunlight or ultraviolet light can trigger a lupus flare.

PATHOGENESIS

B-cell hyper-reactivity leads to the overproduction of auto-antibodies. The primary defect is not known, and there may be different abnormalities leading to loss of B-cell tolerance. One theory is that there is a genetic defect in apoptosis. Apoptotic cells express nuclear antigens on the cell surface where they trigger auto-antibody formation. Auto-antibodies are formed to histones, DNA, RNA; anti-phospholipid antibodies are found in 30% cases. Immune complex deposition and complement activation leads to glomerular damage. The type of glomerular disease depends on the nature of the immune complex (specificity, size, affinity, charge, ability to activate complement) and the rate of its clearance by Fc receptors. Immune complexes cause damage by activating complement, leading to chemokine production and recruitment of inflammatory cells.

CLINICAL HISTORY

Renal involvement usually appears after the initial presentation with SLE, and often follows a chronic remitting and relapsing course. Rarely patients may present with only renal disease and on renal biopsy have diagnostic features of lupus nephritis. Such patients may develop clinical symptoms or serologic tests of active lupus many years after the initial presentation.

Patients with World Health Organization (WHO) class I and II lupus nephritis normally have mild proteinuria and a normal GFR. Patients with WHO class III and IV nephritis typically have an active urinary sediment, heavier proteinuria, hypertension, and reduced GFR. Class V cases usually have nephrotic syndrome as the main presenting syndrome; renal vein thrombosis and pulmonary emboli are common. Over the course of the illness, the histologic pattern may transform from one class to another with associated changes in the clinical features of the renal disease. Rarely patients can present with oligoanuric acute renal failure, and the renal biopsy either shows extensive crescent formation or glomerular capillary thrombi usually associated with anti-phospholipid antibodies.

Lupus tends to flare during pregnancy and the puerperium. The risk is less in females with mild and well-controlled disease. Maternal flares are associated with increased prematurity and fetal mortality.

Systemic lupus erythematosus (SLE) (*continued*)

PHYSICAL EXAMINATION

Patients with lupus nephritis will often have obvious physical signs of SLE, i.e. alopecia, mouth ulcers, skin rash (**69**), Raynaud's phenomenon, non deforming arthritis, and retinal cotton wool spots (**70**).

DIFFERENTIAL DIAGNOSIS

Mild forms of SLE may masquerade as other diseases for many years, especially the joint or neuropsychiatric presentations. Diseases which may be in the differential diagnosis include rheumatoid arthritis, subacute bacterial endocarditis, lymphoma, idiopathic thrombocytopenia, and HIV infection.

INVESTIGATIONS

Anti-nuclear antibodies (ANA) are found in 99% of cases of SLE. They were discovered in the 1940s with the discovery of the LE cell (**71**). The initial screening test for ANAs is the immunofluoresence test; Hep2 cells are incubated with patient's serum and then fluorescein-tagged anti-human gamma globulin is added to produce an apple-green nuclear staining when viewed through the fluorescent microscope. The test is very sensitive, and the pattern of staining may be characteristic for specific antibodies (**72–75**). However, pattern recognition is now replaced with specific assays to identify precisely and quantitate antibody titers.

Anti-dsDNA antibodies are relatively specific (95%) for SLE and often fluctuate with disease activity. In some patients there is no correlation with disease activity. If a patient has been followed for several months and titers correlate with activity, it is likely that titers will continue to be useful for monitoring activity. Anti-dsDNA antibodies may be measured by the Farr assay (ammonium sulphate precipitation), *Crithidia luciliae* assay (**76**) or ELISA. Anti-Smith (anti-Sm) antibodies are directed against small ribonucleoproteins. They are insensitive but highly specific for SLE, and remain so when the disease is inactive and when anti-dsDNA antibodies have fallen into the normal range. They are found in 10–30% of Caucasians and 30–40% of Asians and Afro-Caribbeans with SLE. The presence of anti-Sm antibodies may be associated with milder renal involvement. Ro/SSA and La/SSB antibodies are detected in high frequency in the serum of patients with Sjögren's syndrome and subacute cutaneous lupus and neonatal lupus.

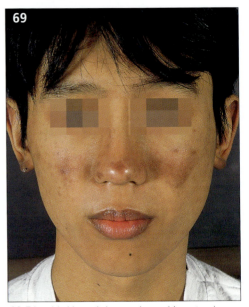

69 Discoid skin rash in a patient with systemic lupus erythematosus.

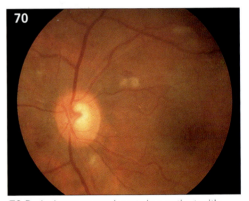

70 Retinal cotton wool spots in a patient with systemic lupus erythematosus.

Many patients with SLE have an activation of the classic complement cascade with consumption of the early complement components C1q, C4, and C3. C4 levels usually fall earlier and to a greater extent than C3 during a disease flare.

Renal biopsy in selected patients is necessary to decide which patients may or may not benefit from immunosuppression.

71 Buffy coat preparation from the peripheral blood of a patient with active lupus showing nuclear material phagocytosed by polymorphs (LE cells) (arrow). Light microscopy (MGG ×1000).

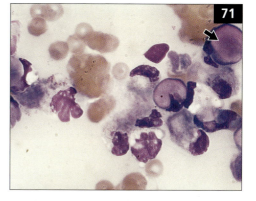

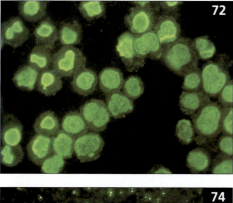

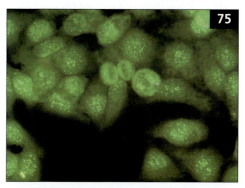

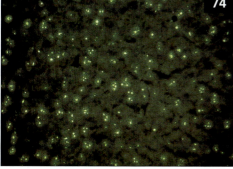

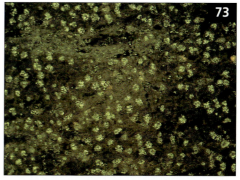

72–76 Different patterns of anti-nuclear antibody staining. Homogeneous staining on Hep2 cells (×1000) (**72**). Speckled pattern on rat liver (×400) (**73**). Nucleolar pattern on rat liver (×400) (**74**). Centromere pattern (×1000) (**75**).

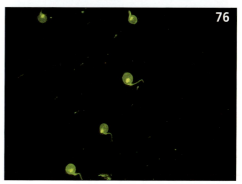

76 Immunofluoresence staining of *Crithidia lucillae*. This trypanosome contains a kinetoplast circular DNA which is double stranded.

Systemic lupus erythematosus (SLE) (*continued*)

HISTOLOGY (77–84)

There is hypercellularity of the glomerular tuft, which can be segmental or global, focal or diffuse, and may include polymorphs. In active disease there may be foci of fibrinoid tuft necrosis, nuclear fragmentation, wire-loops, hyaline thrombi, and crescent formation. Hematoxylin bodies formed from digested nuclear material may be found in areas of necrosis.

Immune deposits are the hallmark of lupus nephritis. A 'full house' of staining for IgG, IgM, IgA, C3, C1q, and C4 is characteristic of lupus nephritis. Mesangial deposits are found even in patients without overt renal disease.

Capillary wall deposits, which are characteristically subendothelial when seen in electron microscopy, cause the thickened, rigid, and refractile capillary wall known as the classic 'wire-loop'. There will often also be subepithelial and intramembranous deposits, which may be an aid to diagnosis. The so-called 'hyaline thrombi' seen in light microscopy are in fact huge subendothelial electron-dense deposits that bulge out into the lumen, sometimes causing occlusion of the glomerular capillary lumen. True thrombi may be seen in the anti-phospholipid syndrome. Rarely, a fingerprint-like pattern or tubuloreticular inclusions may be seen in the electron-dense deposits.

The WHO classification is widely used by nephrologists and renal pathologists:
Class I Normal
Class IIA Mesangial deposits
Class IIB Mesangial hypercellularity
Class III Focal, segmental proliferative
    glomerulonephritis
Class IV Diffuse proliferative glomerulonephritis
Class V Membranous glomerulonephritis

Crescents are commonly found in classes III and IV lupus nephritis. Interstitial nephritis is common and rarely may occur without glomerular involvement. A thrombotic microangiopathy may occur in association with anti-phospholipid antibodies.

Activity indices based on the features mentioned above, and chronicity indices, based on features such as glomerular sclerosis, tubular atrophy, and interstitial fibrosis, are also useful in guiding treatment.

PROGNOSIS

Patient survival has improved in lupus patients over the past few decades. The results from two prospective cohorts of 1000 European and 644 Canadian patients with lupus found 95% and 93% 5-year survival rates, respectively. Most deaths are caused by active SLE, thrombosis, or infection. Renal survival has also improved with the use of cytotoxic drugs.

MANAGEMENT

The management of lupus nephritis is complex. Corticosteroids and azathioprine are used for patients with mild renal involvement. For patients with severe lupus nephritis, intravenous methylprednisolone and cyclophosphamide are necessary but have undesirable side-effects. There is increasing experience with mycophenolate mofetil in the treatment of lupus

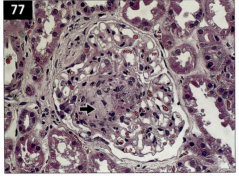

77 Glomerulus from a case of focal proliferative lupus nephritis (WHO class III) showing a segmental area of consolidation and necrosis (arrow). Note the uninvolved tuft is normal. Light microscopy (H+E ×350).

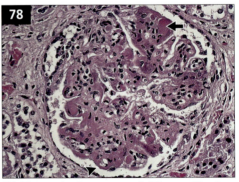

78 Glomerulus from a case of diffuse proliferative lupus nephritis (WHO class IV) showing increased cellularity, wire-loop thickening of capillary walls (arrow head) and hyaline 'thrombi' (arrow). Light microscopy (H+E ×400).

nephritis. Other drugs that have been trialled for lupus nephritis include cyclosporine (cyclosporin), tacrolimus, a thromboxane A2 synthetase inhibitor, anti-CD40 ligand, and anti-interleukin-10. Lupus nephritis recurs infrequently after transplantation.

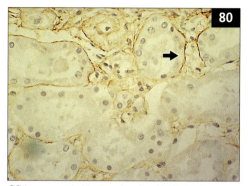

79 Diffuse proliferative lupus nephritis showing IgG localizing on glomerular capillary walls and segmentally in mesangial areas (brown reaction product). Immunoperoxidase (anti-IgG antibody ×400).

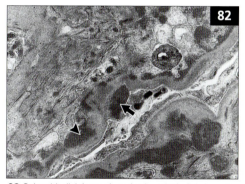

80 Lupus nephritis showing focal IgG staining on tubular basement membranes (brown reaction product, arrow). Immunoperoxidase (anti-IgG antibody ×400).

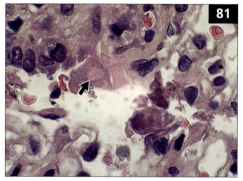

81 Hematoxylin body (arrow). Light microscopy (H+E ×1000).

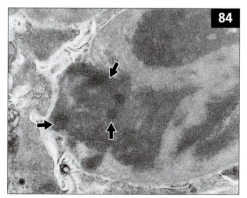

82 Subepithelial (arrow) and subendothelial deposits (arrow head). Electron microscopy (×4000).

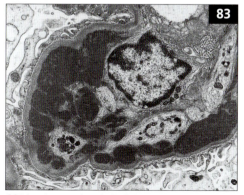

83 Very large subendothelial electron-dense deposits from the same case as **82**, that would equate to the hyaline thrombi seen in light microscopy. Electron microscopy (×5000).

84 High magnification of deposits from the same case as **82**, showing the fingerprint pattern (arrows). Electron microscopy (×10,000).

Primary anti-phospholipid antibody syndrome (PAPS)

DEFINITION
Since the first description of the syndrome in 1981 its protean clinical and laboratory features have been defined. For a positive diagnosis there must be radiologic or histologic evidence of arterial or venous thrombosis, or recurrent miscarriages, and the presence of medium or high titers of IgM or IgG anti-cardiolipin antibodies or lupus anticoagulant on two occasions at least 6 weeks apart. This disorder is referred to as the primary APS when it occurs alone; however, it can also be found in association with SLE, or with certain infections and drugs.

CLINICAL HISTORY
Patients usually have a history of a major thrombotic event such as a deep vein thrombosis or pulmonay emboli. There may be multiple miscarriages or severe pre-eclampsia due to small vessel thrombosis and placental insufficiency. There may be a history of arterial thromboses affecting the cerebral or coronary circulation. Other manifestations include livedo reticularis, hemolytic anemia, thrombocytopenia, neurologic dysfunction, pulmonary hypertension, avascular necrosis, and adrenal failure. Rarely, primary APS can cause multiorgan failure due to multiple small vessel occlusion. Renal involvement may present with hypertension, proteinuria, renal impairment, or acute renal failure. Renal arterial and venous thromboses have been reported. There is an association with renal artery stenosis.

PHYSICAL EXAMINATION
A variety of cutaneous abnormalities may be seen, including livedo reticularis, digital gangrene, and Degos' disease (malignant atrophic papulosis). A major thrombotic event may cause obvious clinical signs.

DIFFERENTIAL DIAGNOSIS
Systemic lupus erythematosus with associated anti-phospholipid antibodies is excluded by the clinical history and a negative ANA. Other thrombophiliac conditions such as Protein C and S deficiency and factor V deficiency should be excluded.

INVESTIGATIONS
The activated partial thromboplastin time is prolonged and is not normalized when the patient's plasma is diluted 1:1 with normal platelet-free plasma (lupus anticoagulant activity). IgG or IgM anti-cardiolipin antibody titers are measured by a standardized ELISA technique. In patients with neurologic involvement there may be multiple, small, high-density lesions on MRI (**85**).

HISTOLOGY
The characterisic pathologic change is a thrombotic microangiopathy with minimal perivascular inflammation (**86**). Renal histological changes include small vessel vaso-occlusive lesions associated with fibrous intimal hyperplasia of interlobular arteries, and focal cortical atrophy.

PROGNOSIS
The renal prognosis is variable but generally the thrombotic microangiopathy leads to progressive renal destruction causing end-stage renal failure and can recur in renal allografts.

MANAGEMENT
Patients with renal involvement must be anticoagulated to keep the INR >3. Selected patients with acute renal failure may respond to plasma exchange and/or immunosuppression.

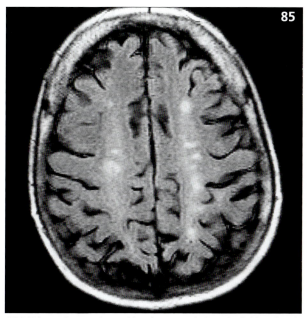

85 MRI scan in a patient with primary anti-phospholipid antibody syndrome demonstrating periventricular white matter lesions.

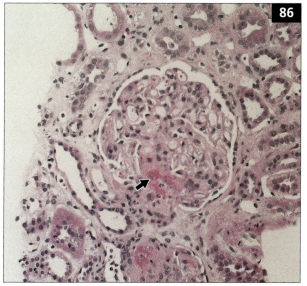

86 Primary anti-phospholipid antibody syndrome. Thrombosis is present within the glomerular tuft and afferent vessels (arrow). Light microscopy (H+E x200).

Systemic vasculitis

DEFINITION

The vasculitides can be classified using only two criteria: the size of the vessel involved and the presence or absence of granuloma formation (*Table 5*).

Large vessel vasculitis is only rarely complicated by glomerulonephritis, and polyarteritis nodosa may cause renal infarction. In renal units small vessel vasculitides are by far the most common type, causing a pauci-immune focal necrotizing and crescentic glomerulonephritis.

EPIDEMIOLOGY AND ETIOLOGY

Small vessel vasculitis is characteristically a disease of middle-aged and elderly patients, with a slight preponderance of males. It can however present in childhood. It is rare in Afro-Caribbean patients. The etiology of systemic vasculitis remains obscure, although a minority of patients may have a bacterial infection, commonly staphylococcal, as a trigger.

PATHOGENESIS

Immune complexes are not found in the glomeruli or vessels of patients with small vessel vasculitis. Cell-mediated immunity involving T-lymphocytes and monocytes is probably critical, as these cells are the predominant types found histologically. The pathogenic role of anti-neutrophil cytoplasmic antibodies (ANCA) remains controversial.

CLINICAL HISTORY

Patients usually present with fever, malaise, and weight loss. Skin, joints, lungs, eyes, and nervous system are commonly affected along with the kidney. Vasculitis may be limited to the kidney; alternatively, in some patients renal involvement may never occur. A diagnosis of Wegener's granulomatosis requires the presence of at least two of the following four criteria: renal involvement, a histologic diagnosis of granulomatous arteritis, an abnormal chest radiograph (**87**), and nasal or oral inflammation.

PHYSICAL EXAMINATION

Arthritis, purpura (**88**), scleritis (**89**), or uveitis may be present. Vasculitic infarcts may be seen commonly in the nail folds, finger pulps, and fundi. Collapse of the bridge of the nose may occur in Wegener's granulomatosis (**90**). Severe hypertension is uncommon.

Table 5 Classification of vasculitis		
	Granulomas	
Size of vessel	*Yes*	*No*
Small	Wegener's granulomatosis	Microscopic polyarteritis Henoch–Schönlein purpura
Medium	Churg–Strauss	Polyarteritis nodosa
Large		Giant cell arteritis Takayasu's syndrome Kawasaki disease

DIFFERENTIAL DIAGNOSIS

Differential diagnoses include atheroembolic disease, infective endocarditis, SLE, and other pulmonary renal syndromes, especially Goodpasture's disease. Patients with the latter condition do not have a skin rash and often do not have the prodromal illness of fever, weight loss, and myalgia that is typical of vasculitis.

INVESTIGATIONS

A normochromic anemia is common, and the platelet count is usually raised. The ESR is invariably raised. Serum albumin is reduced. Microscopic hematuria, proteinuria, and a raised creatinine are usual. The renal function may decline rapidly. Urine microscopy will demonstrate red cell casts. Serum immunoglobulin and complement concentrations are normal. ANCA (**91, 92**) are found in about 90% of untreated cases of small vessel vasculitis. In Wegener's granulomatosis the target is usually a neutrophil granular enzyme proteinase 3 and on immunofluorescence study of ethanol-fixed neutrophils shows a diffuse cytoplasmic staining (c-ANCA pattern). Patients with microscopic polyarteritis generally have p-ANCA which has a perinuclear pattern of staining. The target of p-ANCA is principally myeloperoxidase. ANCA titers can be used to monitor disease activity over time. A renal biopsy is necessary to assess the severity of renal involvement in small vessel vasculitis and thus guide treatment. The value of renal or visceral angiography is minimal in small vessel vasculitis, but diagnostic in cases of large vessel vasculitis.

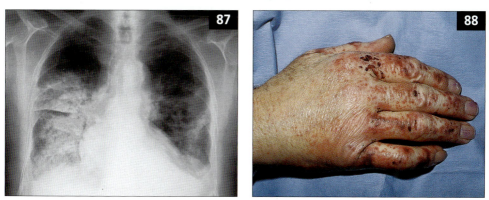

87 Chest radiograph in a patient who presented with ANCA-positive vasculitis, presenting with acute renal failure due to a severe necrotizing glomerulonephritis. The patient subsequently became acutely short of breath with associated hemoptysis. The radiograph shows bilateral diffuse alveolar shadowing due to pulmonary hemorrhage.

88 Vasculitic rash in a patient with rapidly progressive glomerulonephritis (ANCA-positive).

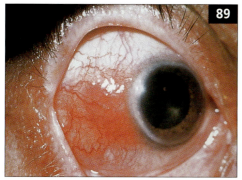

89 Acute focal anterior scleritis in a patient with Wegener's granulomatosis.

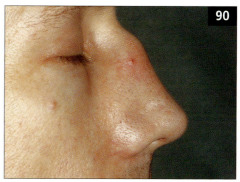

90 A patient with Wegener's granulomatosis showing depression of the bridge of the nose because of involvement of cartilage; the differential diagnosis is relapsing polychondritis.

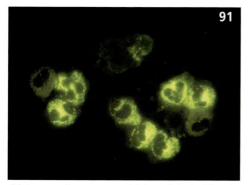

91 Immunofluorescence staining of alcohol-fixed normal human neutrophils. Cytoplasmic (c-ANCA) staining (×1000).

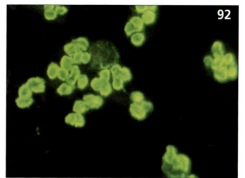

92 Immunofluorescence staining of alcohol-fixed normal human neutrophils. Perinuclear (p-ANCA) staining (×1000).

Systemic vasculitis (*continued*)

HISTOLOGY (93–95)

The typical appearances are dependent on the severity and the length of time the disease has been active. This may be a focal segmental necrotizing glomerulonephritis, with crescent formation or a diffuse global process with 100% crescents. Immunohistochemistry is negative or shows nonspecific segmental localizationof IgM and complement in areas of chronic damage. Fresh necrotizing lesions will show fibrin. Interstitial mononuclear infiltration is common and may be severe, but granulomata are rarely seen in needle biopsies, even in unequivocal clinical Wegener's. Extraglomerular vasculitis is only seen in vessels in a minority of biopsies.

PROGNOSIS

The prognosis for small vessel vasculitis affecting the kidney has improved from almost inevitable death 30 years ago to about 70% 5-year survival currently, with the advent of successful immunosuppressive regimens.

MANAGEMENT

Standard induction treatment involves intravenous methylprednisolone and oral cyclophosphamide. In cases with rapidly deteriorating renal function, plasma exchange is generally used. In resistant cases intravenous immunoglobulin may be used. Maintenance treatment consists of corticosteroids and cyclophosphamide or azathioprine. There is increasing evidence for the use of mycophenolate mofetil as an alternative maintenance agent.

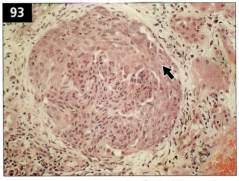

93 A glomerular tuft showing fibrinoid necrosis and surrounded by a circumferential crescent (arrow). Light microscopy (H+E ×400).

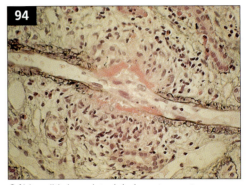

94 Vasculitis in an interlobular artery cut longitudinally. There is a dense local mononuclear cell infiltrate. Light microscopy (H+E ×400).

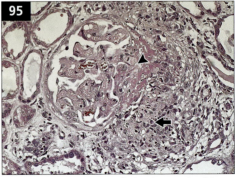

95 A glomerulus showing fibrinoid necrosis of the arteriole at the hilum (arrow head) and an adjacent granuloma (arrow) in a patient with Wegener's granulomatosis. Light microscopy (H+E ×350).

Sickle cell anemia and glomerulonephritis

DEFINITION
Sickle cell disease (homozygous hemoglobin SS) and sickle cell trait (heterozygous hemoglobin SA) are associated with a variety of renal abnormalities including impaired concentration of the urine leading to polyuria, hematuria, papillary necrosis, acute renal failure related to multiple organ failure during a sickle cell crisis, and glomerulonephritis causing nephrotic syndrome and end-stage renal failure.

EPIDEMIOLOGY AND ETIOLOGY
The incidence of proteinuria in patients with sickle cell disease is common. End-stage renal disease has been reported in 10–20% of adults with sickle cell disease. This proportion is likely to increase with improved survival due to better medical treatment of other complications of this condition.

PATHOGENESIS
The chronic anemia leads to increased renal blood flow and glomerular filtration rate. This leads to the increased glomerular size, and later to focal and segmental glomerulosclerosis. Other factors may play a role including iron overload, debris from erythrocytes phagocytosed by glomeruli, and immune complexes. Medullary hypoxia leads to sickling and damage to the urine-concentrating mechanism.

HISTOLOGY
Focal and segmental glomerulosclerosis is the commonest lesion. A mesangiocapillary glomerulonephritis can also occur (96).

PROGNOSIS
Patients with glomerulosclerosis progress over months or years to end-stage renal failure.

MANAGEMENT
ACE inhibitors may prolong renal survival. Renal transplantation has been performed successfully in this condition.

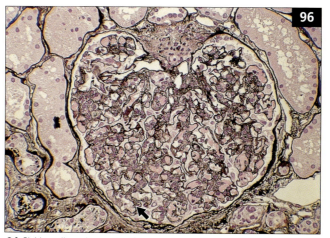

96 Sickle cell nephropathy. Glomerular capillary wall shows double-contouring (arrow). Light microscopy (MS x250).

Goodpasture's disease

DEFINITION

Goodpasture's disease is caused by anti-basement membrane antibody production, leading to glomerular and pulmonary injury. Patients may have severe pulmonary hemorrhage and only minor renal involvement; alternatively, they may have severe renal involvement and no lung involvement, or severe pulmonary and renal disease.

EPIDEMIOLOGY AND ETIOLOGY

Goodpasture's disease is a rare disease occurring in about 0.5 cases/million/year. It is associated with HLA-DR2. Cigarette smoking and exposure to organic solvents and hydrocarbons have been implicated with cases of this disease. There have been case reports of the condition associated with membranous glomerulonephritis, lymphoma, and lithotripsy.

PATHOGENESIS

The pathogenic anti-glomerular basement membrane antibody (anti-GBM) is directed against the noncollagenous NC1 domain of the $\alpha3(IV)$-chain of basement membrane collagen. Although this is the archetypal antibody-mediated disease, there is also clear involvement of T-cells in its pathogenesis.

CLINICAL HISTORY

The prodromal symptoms of malaise, weight loss, and arthralgia are less marked than in systemic vasculitis. Renal impairment at presentation is usually severe, and deteriorates rapidly. Macroscopic hematuria and loin pain may occur. Pulmonary hemorrhage occurs in about two-thirds of patients. The amount of hemoptysis correlates poorly with the severity of hemorrhage. Pulmonary hemorrhage can remit and relapse and there may be a history of episodic breathlessness over the previous months.

PHYSICAL EXAMINATION

It may be difficult to distinguish clinically and radiologically between respiratory failure due to pulmonary edema secondary to renal failure and pulmonary hemorrhage.

DIFFERENTIAL DIAGNOSIS

The other principal causes of rapidly progressive glomerulonephritis with alveolar hemorrhage include systemic vasculitis and SLE. The main differential diagnoses of acute renal and respiratory failure are pulmonary edema due to fluid overload in acute renal failure, opportunistic infections in patients with rapidly progressive glomerulonephritis who have been heavily immunosuppressed, severe cardiac failure, and paraquat poisoning.

INVESTIGATIONS

Anti-GBM IgG auto-antibodies are detected by ELISA, radioimmunoassay, or indirect immunofluorescence. Monitoring anti-GBM levels is helpful in guiding the intensity of treatment. In about 10% of cases ANCA titers are positive and these patients tend to have features of systemic vasculitis. Measurement of the rate of carbon monoxide uptake by the lung (K_{CO}) is helpful in distinguishing between pulmonary hemorrhage and pulmonary edema.

HISTOLOGY (97, 98)

A renal biopsy is essential for prognostic purposes. In cases with severe renal involvement there is a diffuse, extracapillary, proliferative glomerulonephritis, with necrosis and extensive crescent formation. There may be rupture of Bowman's capsule. There is usually an interstitial nephritis. Immunohistochemistry shows linear localization of IgG and frequently C3 on the glomerular capillary basement membrane.

PROGNOSIS

Patients with severe renal impairment (>70% crescents and plasma creatinine >600 μmol/l [6.8 mg/dl]) have a poor renal prognosis. Patients with less severe disease may respond to immunosuppression. Recurrence of renal or respiratory disease is a rare but recognized phenomenon. Renal transplantation should be postponed until at least 6 months after the disappearance of circulating anti-GBM antibodies.

MANAGEMENT

Induction treatment consists of plasma exchange to remove the pathogenic antibody and immunosuppression with corticosteroids and cyclophosphamide. Immunosuppression can usually be stopped after 3 months.

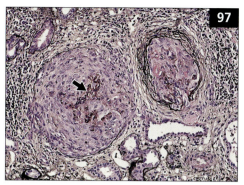

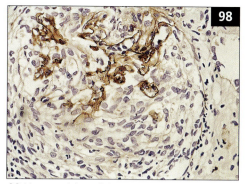

97 Two glomeruli in anti-GBM disease showing occlusive cellular crescents. The residual silver positive glomerular tuft is shown (arrow). Light microscopy (MS x250).

98 Linear staining of the glomerular capillary walls with IgG (brown reaction product). Immunoperoxidase (anti-IgG antibody x400).

Glomerulonephritis associated with hepatitis B virus infection

DEFINITION

Hepatitis B virus infection is associated with two major forms of renal involvement: polyarteritis nodosa and membranous glomerulonephritis.

PATHOGENESIS

Hepatitis B-associated membranous glomerulonephritis is probably immune complex-mediated. HBsAg, HBcAg and HBeAg have all been identified in the glomeruli, but it is thought that the HBeAg or antigen–antibody complex are the appropriate size and charge to cross the glomerular basement membrane and deposit in the subepithelial space.

CLINICAL HISTORY

Patients with hepatitis B-associated membranous glomerulonephritis usually present with nephrotic syndrome. At presentation most patients have a normal serum creatinine but often massive proteinuria. Liver involvement is usually mild at the time of renal presentation, with a normal bilirubin and modestly raised values for serum alanine aminotransferase levels. Liver biopsy usually shows mild chronic active hepatitis rather than cirrhosis.

HISTOLOGY

The light microscopic appearances are similar to idiopathic membranous glomerulonephritis, except there may be more mesangial cell proliferation and there may be areas of focal mesangiocapillary change in some of the capillary loops. All cases stain for IgG, and most for IgM and complement. A subset of patients have mesangial IgA deposits. HBsAg and HBcAg are found inconsistently in the glomeruli, whereas HBeAg is commonly found in subepithelial deposits.

PROGNOSIS

Most children clear HBsAg from the blood with resolution of proteinuria without residual renal impairment. This course is rare in adults and there is usually progression to renal failure over months to years.

MANAGEMENT

Symptoms associated with nephrotic syndrome are treated with salt restriction, diuretics, and lipid lowering agents. Corticosteroids may enhance viral replication and worsen the liver and renal disease. Interferon has been successful at reducing viral replication, clearing HBsAg from the blood, and reducing proteinuria in some patients.

Glomerulonephritis associated with hepatitis C virus infection

DEFINITION
Patients with hepatitis C infection may develop mesangiocapillary glomerulonephritis or cryoglobulinemic glomerulonephritis.

EPIDEMIOLOGY AND ETIOLOGY
Hepatitis C is a blood-borne virus transmitted sexually, by blood transfusion, and by sharing needles for intravenous drug use or tattooing. Areas of high prevalence of infection include North America, southern Europe, and the Indian subcontinent.

PATHOGENESIS
Hepatitis C infection can lead to chronic active hepatitis, cirrhosis, and hepatoma. Mixed essential cryoglobulins are commonly found and contain HCV RNA and anti-HCV IgG. The mechanisms that trigger precipitation of cryoglobulins within the glomeruli are not known, but once in the glomeruli they bind complement and induce chemokine production leading to inflammatory cell recruitment.

CLINICAL HISTORY AND PHYSICAL EXAMINATION
Patients usually have symptoms and signs of chronic liver disease. The renal disease may present with proteinuria, microscopic hematuria, nephrotic syndrome, or renal impairment. Patients may develop a purpuric rash (**99**) or arthralgias. Hypertension may be severe.

DIFFERENTIAL DIAGNOSIS
ANCA-positive vasculitis presenting with a rash and renal impairment is distinguished by the presence of ANCA serologically and renal biopsy appearances. Type 1 cryoglobulins are monoclonal immunoglobulins found in multiple myeloma, Waldenstrom's macroglobulinemia, or benign monoclonal gammopathy.

INVESTIGATIONS
Cryoglobulinemia is usually associated with low C3 and C4 levels. Cryocrits are variable and correlate poorly with the disease activity. Anti-HCV IgG is detected by ELISA and HCV RNA by PCR.

HISTOLOGY (100–102)
The light microscopic appearances are of diffuse intracapillary hypercellularity, often severe enough to occlude the capillary lumina. The hypercellularity consists of a mixture of resident glomerular cells, and migrating neutrophils, T-cells and especially monocytes. Eosinophilic thrombi are often found in the capillary lumina and consist of cryoprecipitable immunoglobulins. Immunohistochemistry shows localization of IgG and IgM in these areas. Electron microscopy shows dense subendothelial deposits which may occlude the glomerular capillary. High magnification often reveals a microtubular appearance which may show a curved annular and cylindric configuration. Vasculitis affecting small or medium sized arteries may be seen in patients with an acute clinical picture.

PROGNOSIS
The clinical course is very variable but progression to end-stage renal failure is rare. Death is more commonly due to nonrenal complications such as vasculitis, hypertension, and infections.

MANAGEMENT
Combination treatment with interferon and ribavirin can clear the virus from the circulation, although replication often recurs after stopping the antiviral agents. Antiviral drugs have been shown to improve liver histology. Plasma exchange may be used if there is evidence of severe acute nephritis or evidence of a systemic vasculitis.

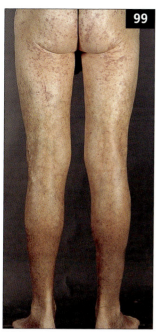

99 Purpuric rash in a patient with chronic hepatitis C infection and cryoglobulinemia.

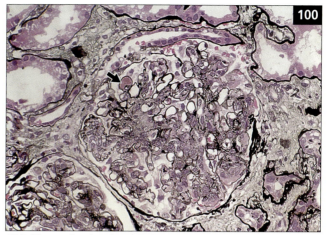

100 Glomerulus showing global increase of cellularity, mesangial expansion, and an eosinophilic 'thrombus' (arrow). Light microscopy (MS x250).

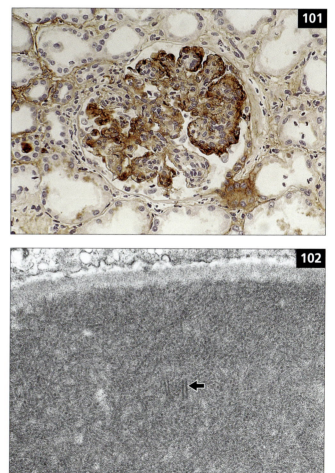

101 Glomerulus showing peripheral capillary wall localization of IgM (brown reaction product). Immunoperoxidase (anti-IgM antibody x250).

102 Microtubule formation. Electron microscopy (x10,000).

Glomerulonephritis associated with human immunodeficiency virus (HIV)

DEFINITION

HIV infection can cause renal complications in many ways. Electrolyte, acid–base disorders and acute renal failure may occur, often due to sepsis from opportunistic infections or related to chemotherapy for neoplasia. HUS/TTP is a recognized complication of HIV infection. Almost all types of glomerular lesions have been reported in HIV-seropositive patients. However, the characteristic glomerular lesion is a collapsing form of focal and segmental glomerulonephritis. This human immunodeficiency virus-associated nephropathy (HIVAN) is the subject of this section.

EPIDEMIOLOGY AND ETIOLOGY

HIVAN is much more common in blacks than whites (about 10:1). The reasons for this are not known, although an increased susceptibility of blacks to renal disease is seen with the increased frequency in blacks of hypertensive nephrosclerosis, diabetic renal disease, and idiopathic focal and segmental glomerulosclerosis. HIVAN can present before there has been any other AIDS-defining illness.

PATHOGENESIS

Experiments using transgenic mice expressing certain HIV proteins provide strong evidence that direct infection of renal cells by the virus leads to production of inflammatory cytokines, thus leading to development of HIVAN. Host genetic factors are also important.

CLINICAL HISTORY AND PHYSICAL EXAMINATION

Patients usually present with nephrotic range proteinuria and renal impairment. The presence of hypertension is variable. Edema is often minimal. There may be physical signs suggesting HIV infection, e.g. hairy leucoplakia, herpetic lesions, or Kaposi's sarcoma.

DIFFERENTIAL DIAGNOSIS

Patients with heroin-associated nephropathy usually have small kidneys on ultrasound, a noncollapsing focal and segmental glomerulonephritis, and a slow progression to end-stage renal failure.

INVESTIGATIONS

Renal ultrasound in HIVAN characteristically shows abnormally large echo-bright kidneys (**103**). HIV serology is positive and there is usually a reduction in the CD4 count.

HISTOLOGY (104–106)

There are a number of different renal histological characteristic changes in the glomeruli and tubules. There may be a focal and segmental collapsing glomerulopathy with shrinkage and sclerosis of the entire glomerulus, leaving Bowman's space empty or filled with acidophilic proteinaceous material. There may alternatively be a marked proliferation of glomerular epithelial cells such that the appearances mimic a cellular crescent. Another form of renal involvement is a striking focal microcystic dilatation of renal tubules which are filled with casts. There may also be an interstitial nephritis. Immunohistochemistry may show nonspecific localizationof IgM and C3 in the mesangium and sclerotic areas. Electron-dense deposits may be found in the mesangium. Tubuloreticular inclusions are commonly found in endothelial cells.

PROGNOSIS

Untreated, there is rapid progression to end-stage renal failure over a matter of weeks or months.

MANAGEMENT

ACE inhibitors reduce proteinuria and slow the progression to end-stage renal failure. Treatment with combination antiretroviral therapy has led to stabilization or improvement in renal function in patients with HIVAN. It is thus important to make a diagnosis of HIVAN as progression to renal failure can be stopped with antiviral drugs.

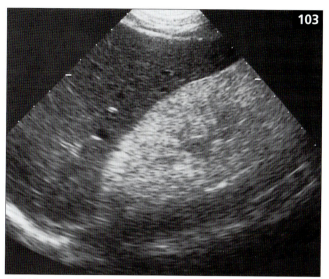

103 Ultrasound demonstrating large echogenic kidneys.

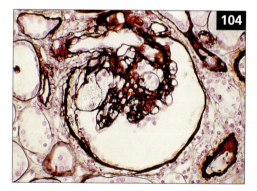

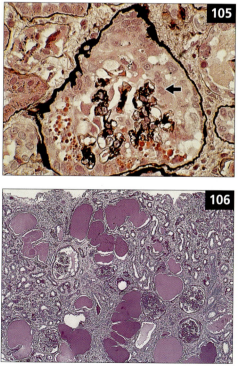

104 Glomerulus showing collapsed shrunken tuft (collapsing FSGS). Light microscopy (MS ×400).

105 Glomerulus showing severe proliferation of epithelial cells in Bowman's space mimicking a crescent (arrow). Light microscopy (MS ×400).

106 Cortical tubules showing focal cystic dilatation with eosinophilic casts. Light microscopy (PAS ×150).

Miscellaneous infections and glomerulonephritis

SYPHILIS

The commonest glomerular lesion is membranous nephropathy. Fine granular deposits of IgG, IgM, and C3 are found in the capillary wall and mesangium. Spirochetes may be seen on light microscopy in the interstitium and tubules. Treponemal antigen and antibody have been found and it is thought to be an immune complex nephropathy. Proteinuria usually resolves after penicillin treatment.

LEPROSY

The major renal lesions are glomerulonephritis and secondary amyloidosis. Morphologically, the commonest types of glomerular lesions are mesangial proliferative and diffuse proliferative glomerulonephritis. Granular deposits of IgG and C3 are seen in the mesangium and capillary wall. Electron microscopy demonstrates subepithelial and subendothelial deposits. Amyloidosis is much more common in lepromatous than tuberculoid leprosy. There is no convincing evidence that antileprosy drugs alter the course of the glomerular lesions.

SCHISTOSOMIASIS

Schistosoma hematobium which is widely prevalent in the Middle East and Africa does not cause glomerulonephritis but affects the ureters and bladder which can lead to obstructive uropathy. *Schistosoma mansoni* which is prevalent in Brazil, Egypt, and east Africa causes an immune complex-mediated disease. It usually presents in patients with hepatosplenic disease with nephrotic syndrome. Serum complement levels are low and circulating immune complexes may be found. In early disease mesangial proliferation or mesangiocapillary nephropathy are found. Focal and segmental glomerulosclerosis and amyloid deposits may also be found. IgG, IgE, IgM, and less often IgA and C3 are found in the capillary walls and mesangium. Progression to end-stage renal failure is over several years, and is not affected by antiparasitic drugs or immunosuppression.

MALARIA

Plasmodium falciparum can cause a mild mesangial proliferative glomerulonephritis which completely resolves after antimalarial treatment. Severe falciparum malaria is associated with intravascular hemolysis and acute renal failure (blackwater fever), with acute tubular necrosis. *Plasmodium malariae* (quartan malaria) is a common cause of nephrotic syndrome in west and east Africa. The patient may present with mild proteinuria or nephrotic syndrome with massive edema and ascites. The disease progresses slowly, leading to hypertension and renal failure within 3–5 years. The renal disease does not respond to steroids or antimalarial treatment. In early cases there is focal and segmental thickening of the capillary walls, which may be double-contoured (**107**). Later the capillary walls become occluded and there is diffuse mesangial sclerosis. There are granular deposits of IgG and IgM along the capillary walls.

MALIGNANCY AND GLOMERULONEPHRITIS

Neoplastic disorders can affect the kidneys in various ways. Leukemia or lymphoma can cause diffuse infiltration of both kidneys causing acute renal failure. Malignancy in the retroperitoneum or lower urinary tract can cause obstructive uropathy. However, tumors are also associated with various forms of glomerulonephritis which resolve on eradication of the tumor. Lymphoma can be associated with minimal change disease. Membranous glomerulonephritis is associated with carcinomas of the lung, stomach, breast, ovary, cervix, and thyroid. Crescentic glomerulonephritis can occur rarely in patients with malignancy. Secondary amyloidosis can be associated with renal cell carcinoma.

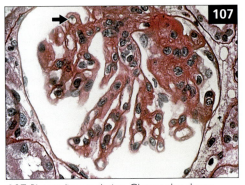

107 *Plasmodium malariae.* Glomerulus shows mesangial sclerosis and segmental double-contouring of the capillary wall (arrow). Light microscopy (PAS x400).

Chapter Four

Tubulointerstitial diseases

- **Acute interstitial nephritis (AIN)**

- **Granulomatous interstitial nephritis**

- **Urate nephropathy**

- **Lead nephropathy**

- **Lithium-induced renal disease**

- **Radiation nephritis**

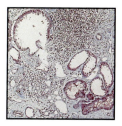
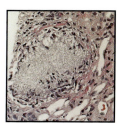
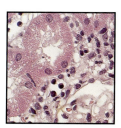
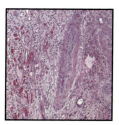

Acute interstitial nephritis (AIN)

DEFINITION
AIN is an acute, usually reversible, inflammatory disease, characterized by the presence of a mononuclear cellular infiltrate within the renal interstitium.

EPIDEMIOLOGY AND ETIOLOGY
AIN is a relatively common cause of acute renal dysfunction comprising approximately 10–15% of cases of acute renal failure in large reported series. It can occur in any age group, but is rare in children. AIN is most frequently associated with drugs, particularly antibiotic, or nonsteroidal anti-inflammatory drugs. Infections are the second most common cause of AIN. AIN also occurs in association with selected autoimmune systemic diseases, and malignancies. In 10–20% of cases, AIN is idiopathic (*Table 6*).

PATHOGENESIS
AIN is considered an immune-mediated allergic reaction triggered against an inciting (renal or extrarenal) antigen. Potential mechanisms include binding of the antigen to kidney membranes, acting as haptens, or formation of circulating immune complexes with deposition in the kidney. In humans, a T-cell-mediated mechanism is suggested by the predominance of T-cell lymphocytes in the interstitial infiltrates, and the general absence of antibody deposition in tubules or interstitium. T-cell reactivity against the antigen (drug) has been demonstrated *in vitro*, using standard lymphocyte stimulation assays. An antibody-mediated mechanism cannot, however, be excluded. In some patients with drug-induced AIN, renal biopsies will show IgG and complement deposition along the tubular basement membrane. Anti-tubular basement membrane antibody is also present in some cases. In addition, IgE antibodies to the drug have been demonstrated in several patients. It is possible that different immunologic mechanisms operate to varying degrees in different patients. When AIN is secondary to a drug, the response is idiosyncratic and unrelated to drug dosage.

CLINICAL HISTORY
Presentation is acute, with oliguria present in approximately 40% of cases. In patients with drug-induced AIN, systemic manifestations of a hypersensitivity reaction include fever (50%), maculopapular rash (40%), and arthralgias (10%). Flank pain is secondary to distension of the renal capsule and occurs in approximately

Table 6 Common causes of acute interstitial nephritis

Drugs
- Antibiotics: penicillin G, ampicillin, methicillin, rifampin (rifampicin), ciprofloxacin, sulfonamides (sulphonamides), trimethoprim + sulfamethoxazole (co-trimoxazole)
- Nonsteroidal anti-inflammatory drugs
- Phenytoin
- Allopurinol
- Diuretics (thiazides, furosemide [frusemide])
- Cimetidine, ranitidine
- Propylthiouracil
- Phenindione

Infectious agents
- Bacteria: *Legionella, Brucella, Streptococcus, Staphylococcus, Pneumococcus*
- Virus: Epstein–Barr, CMV, Hanta virus, HIV, hepatitis B, polyoma virus
- Fungal: *Candida, Histoplasma*
- Parasites: malaria, *Toxoplasma, Schistosoma, Leishmania*

Systemic diseases
- Systemic lupus erythematosus
- Sjögren's syndrome
- Sarcoidosis
- Mixed cryoglobulinemia
- Wegener's granulomatosis

Others
- Herbal medicines (aristolochia fangchi)

Idiopathic

50% of the cases. Hematuria is common but is rarely macroscopic. Renal impairment can vary from a mild elevation in serum creatinine to severe acute renal failure requiring dialysis. Tubular damage can impair the urinary concentration mechanism and result in the development of polyuria. Tubular dysfunction can be also manifested by the development of a renal tubular acidosis (RTA) with both type I (distal) and type II (proximal) RTA occurring.

PHYSICAL EXAMINATION
Low-grade fever and a maculopapular rash may be present. Mild arthralgias are common, but arthritis is unusual.

DIFFERENTIAL DIAGNOSIS

The presence of an intense infiltrate of lymphocytes and eosinophils clearly distinguishes AIN from acute ischemic or nephrotoxic injury. Fever, lumbar pain, and leukocyturia are seen in patients with acute pyelonephritis, but in this condition bacteriuria and leukocytosis are also present, and renal biopsy will show focal areas of infiltrating neutrophils. In chronic forms of interstitial nephritis secondary to drugs (analgesic nephropathy, lithium, gold), interstitial fibrosis and tubular atrophy are prominent, with fewer eosinophils present. Sarcoidosis, Sjögren's syndrome, systemic lupus erythematosus, and mixed cryoglobulinemia may all present as AIN, and need to be considered in the diagnosis. Interstitial infiltrates by atypical and monomorphic cells can be seen in leukemia or lymphoma.

INVESTIGATIONS

Eosinophilia is common (40%). Urinalysis demonstrates hematuria, sterile pyuria, and white blood cell casts in over 75% of the cases. Rarely, red blood cell casts can be seen in the urinary sediment. The presence of eosinophiluria (>1%), observed better with Hansel's stain, is suggestive of AIN but is also seen in other unrelated renal pathologies. The absence of eosinophiluria should never discourage the diagnosis. Proteinuria is generally mild (<1 g/24 h). Serologic markers are usually normal except when AIN is part of a systemic autoimmune process (e.g. SLE). On ultrasound, kidneys appear normal or slightly increased in size.

HISTOLOGY

Because of the poor predictive value of clinical criteria, the diagnosis of AIN requires a renal biopsy. On light microscopy, there is a marked inflammatory interstitial infiltrate and interstitial edema, most commonly involving the deep cortex and outer medulla (108). The interstitial infiltrate is predominantly made up of CD4+ T-cell lymphocytes, but monocytes, eosinophils, and plasma cells can also be present. In severe cases, there is disruption of the tubular basement membrane and the presence of tubulitis. Glomeruli and vessels are usually spared. Glomerular involvement producing a minimal change lesion is seen with the use of NSAIDs. Occasionally, interstitial granulomas can be seen, especially in cases of drug-induced AIN. Both immunofluorescence and electron microscopy are usually negative. Occasionally, a linear or granular staining for IgG or complement may be seen along the tubular basement membrane.

PROGNOSIS

Historically, drug-induced AIN has been considered a reversible process with renal function returning to baseline in the majority of patients. However, recent studies have shown that impaired renal function can persist long-term in up to 40% of the patients. Predictors of poor outcome include the presence of diffuse infiltrates, interstitial fibrosis, tubular atrophy, and granuloma formation on renal biopsy. Additional factors that correlate with a poor outcome include pre-existing impaired renal failure and persistence of oliguria (>3 weeks).

MANAGEMENT

Therapy is primarily supportive. The likely inciting factor(s) need to be identified and eliminated. In patients with drug-induced AIN, available data from small, uncontrolled, retrospective series suggest that treatment with corticosteroids may hasten the recovery of renal function, and may be of benefit in patients who fail to regain renal function within 1 week of stopping the offending agent. To date, no prospective, randomized, well-controlled clinical trial has assessed the role of corticosteroid therapy in patients with drug-induced AIN. Corticosteroids are not indicated in infection-related AIN. In patients with AIN associated with autoimmune systemic diseases, steroid treatment may result in dramatic improvement of renal function.

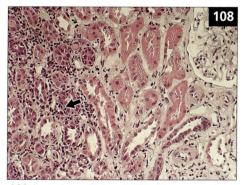

108 Acute interstitial nephritis with mononuclear cells infiltrating tubules (arrow). Light microscopy (H+E ×150).

Granulomatous interstitial nephritis

DEFINITION
Granulomatous interstitial nephritis encompasses a subset of cases of acute interstitial nephritis in which granulomas are present in the interstitium. A granuloma is an inflammatory reaction characterized by the accumulation and proliferation of various cell types, but mainly macrophages. Giant cells are often found as well.

EPIDEMIOLOGY AND ETIOLOGY
The presence of granulomas in renal biopsies is rare. In large renal biopsy series in which interstitial nephritis is the predominant change, granulomas are found in only 1–5% of cases.

> ### Table 7 Recognized causes of granulomatous interstitial nephritis
>
> *Drugs*
> - Antibiotics: penicillin G, ampicillin, methicillin, oxacillin, ciprofloxacin, rifampin (rifampicin), nitrofurantoin, sulfonamides (sulphonamides), trimethoprim + sulfamethoxazole (co-trimoxazole), spiramycin
> - Nonsteroidal anti-inflammatory drugs
> - Anticonvulsants: phenytoin, lamotrigine, carbamazepine
> - Diuretics: furosemide (frusemide), hydrochlorothiazide, triamterene
> - Others: allopurinol, glafenine (glafenin), captopril, cimetidine, fenofibrate, phenindione, acyclovir (aciclovir)
>
> *Infections*
> - Bacteria: *Mycobacteria* (*tuberculosis, kansasii, leprae*), *Brucella, Salmonella,* Whipple's
> - Virus: Epstein–Barr
> - Fungi: *Histoplasma, Candida*
> - Parasites: *Toxoplasma, Schistosoma*
>
> *Foreign body reaction*
> - Oxalate, uric acid
>
> *TINU (tubulointerstitial nephritis–uveitis syndrome)*
>
> *Others*
> - Crohn's, sarcoidosis, Wegener's granulomatosis, heroin use
>
> *Idiopathic*

Drug reactions are the most likely cause of acute granulomatous interstitial nephritis. Drugs most commonly associated with causing granulomatous interstitial nephritis are antibiotics, nonsteroidal anti-inflammatory agents, and diuretics. Besides drugs, other agents or disease processes recognized in association with granulomatous interstitial nephritis include infections, autoimmune diseases and foreign body reactions. In some instances, no etiologic factor can be identified and the condition is called idiopathic.

PATHOGENESIS
The pathogenic mechanism is poorly understood. Proposed immunologic mechanisms include: T-cell-mediated delayed hypersensitivity, anti-tubular basement membrane antibodies, and reaginic antibodies.

CLINICAL HISTORY
The great majority of patients present with acute renal failure. Anuria is not uncommon. As with other patients with an AIN, a maculopapular rash may be present, accompanied by eosinophilia. Other signs and symptoms may reflect the underlying pathogenic process.

PHYSICAL EXAMINATION
As with patients with AIN, low-grade fever and a maculopapular rash may be present. Patients with granulomatous interstitial nephritis secondary to a systemic illness may have characteristic signs of the disease (e.g. erythema nodosum in a patient with sarcoidosis).

DIFFERENTIAL DIAGNOSIS
Granulomatous interstitial nephritis has been described in association with a number of clinical conditions as listed in *Table 7*.

INVESTIGATIONS
In cases of sarcoidosis, serum angiotensin converting enzyme (ACE) levels are usually raised, and a gallium scan will characteristically show increased uptake in the parotid glands, hilar regions of the lungs, and the kidneys.

HISTOLOGY (109, 110)
The number of interstitial granulomas varies greatly from case to case. Typically, granulomas form a nodular infiltrate comparable in size to a glomerulus. The cellular infiltrate is formed mainly of mononuclear cells. Macrophages are the principal elements in a granuloma, but

lymphocytes, plasma cells, and fibroblasts are also found. Epithelioid cells tend to cluster together at the periphery of the nodule. Giant multinuclear cells are occasionally observed. Necrosis may occur at the center of the granuloma, depending on its cause (e.g. tuberculosis). Granulomas are accompanied by an intense lymphocytic interstitial infiltrate. Immunofluorescence shows no deposition of immunoglobulins or complement.

PROGNOSIS

In patients with acute granulomatous interstitial nephritis, prognosis is usually good. In some cases, renal function will recover slowly over a period of months, while others will have persistent renal insufficiency long term.

MANAGEMENT

Treatment will depend on the causative factor. In patients with a drug-induced nephritis, removal of the inciting agent is imperative. Corticosteroids are commonly used and may hasten the recovery of renal function. Corticosteroids are indicated in cases where granulomatous interstitial nephritis is associated with systemic diseases (e.g. sarcoidosis). In infection-associated cases, treatment is targeted to the underlying infection. In patients with tuberculosis-induced granulomatous interstitial nephritis, there have been reports of successful treatment with combined antituberculous drugs and corticosteroids.

109, 110 Interstitial nephritis (carbamazepine-induced) showing a granuloma with associated mononuclear cells and a multinucleate giant cell (arrow). Light microscopy. Low power (H+E ×100) (**109**). High power (H+E ×250) (**110**).

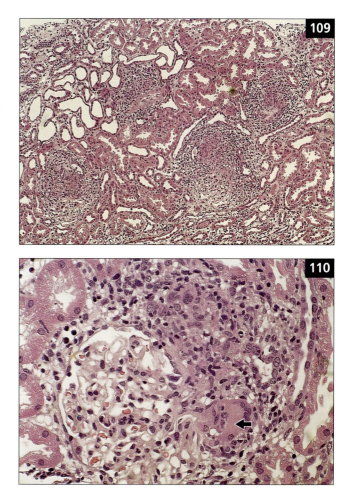

Urate nephropathy

DEFINITION
There are mainly three forms of renal presentation by which pathologic alterations in uric acid metabolism or excretion may occur: acute uric acid nephropathy, chronic uric acid nephropathy, and uric acid stones.

EPIDEMIOLOGY AND ETIOLOGY
Until approximately 40 years ago, renal failure appeared to have been a common complication of middle-aged males with gout. Nowadays, however, the presence of renal failure in patients with 'primary' or classic gout is rare. Relatively recent studies have shown that, in patients with gout, renal function is almost always normal for their age and in the absence of hypertension remains stable over time. The reason for this historic discrepancy is unclear, but it may reflect better control of hyperuricemia after introduction of allopurinol.

PATHOGENESIS
Uric acid is the final degradation product of purine metabolism in humans. Approximately two-thirds of the daily turnover of uric acid is excreted in the urine through a complex process involving glomerular filtration, proximal tubule absorption and secretion, and further reabsorption along the proximal renal tubule. Urate clearance is affected by a number of factors including the extracellular volume, urinary flow rate, acid–base balance, urinary pH, and plasma urate levels.

Acute hyperuricemic nephropathy
Acute hyperuricemic nephropathy is an important cause of oliguric acute renal failure. It is said to occur in up to 5% of patients with myeloproliferative disorders or neoplasias, especially while undergoing chemotherapy or radiation (tumor lysis syndrome). Other conditions associated with sudden cell lysis and rapid increase in serum uric acid levels include hemolysis and rhabdomyolysis. These pathologic situations are usually associated with an increase in purine catabolism, resulting in markedly increased uric acid levels in the serum and massive uricosuria. Risk factors for acute hyperuricemic nephropathy include dehydration, low urinary volume, high serum uric acid levels, urinary pH <5.0, rapid response to chemotherapy, pre-existing renal failure, and use of radiocontrast dye, all of which markedly increase uric acid excretion. In these settings, uric acid levels reach supersaturation values in the urine and uric acid crystallizes within the tubular lumen. Crystallization occurs predominantly in the medullary collecting ducts, resulting in the development of tubular obstruction and acute renal failure.

Chronic uric acid nephropathy
Chronic uric acid nephropathy is thought to result from the deposition of monosodium urate crystals in the renal interstitium, but its pathogenesis is controversial. The frequent co-existence of hypertension, hyperlipidemia, atherosclerotic vascular disease, and diabetes (all conditions that by themselves can cause renal injury) in patients with gout has led some investigators to suggest that the progressive renal failure seen in these patients is primarily a result of the above conditions, rather than secondary to abnormalities in uric acid handling. How the uric acid crystals reach the renal interstitium is equally controversial. In experimental models of crystal-induced nephropathies, the initial event includes damage to the tubular epithelium, disruption of the basement membrane, with migration of crystals into the interstitium. This is followed by phagocytosis of uric acid crystals by polymorphonuclear leukocytes, leukocyte degranulation, and lysis of adjacent cellular components, resulting in the formation of renal microtophi and development of an inflammatory response in the form of a chronic interstitial nephritis. Urate crystal may also injure cells directly by forming hydrogen bonds with the cellular membrane. In these experiments, even short periods of crystal deposition resulted in severe renal damage. Although deposited crystals eventually disappear, progressive renal failure continues.

CLINICAL HISTORY
Acute hyperuricemic nephropathy classically occurs in the setting of a 'tumor lysis syndrome'. It typically presents with a history of acute oliguria in a patient with leukemia or lymphoma who has recently (within 48 hours) been treated with cytotoxic therapy. In this situation, massive cell lysis results in hyperkalemia, hyperphosphatemia, hypocalcemia, and acidosis. Metabolic abnormalities develop quickly, and uric acid levels can rise to 15–20 mg/dl (0.9–1.2 mmol/l), with massive uricosuria. In the acidic milieu of the collecting tubules, uric acid crystallizes, causing acute tubular obstruction, oliguria, and azotemia.

Chronic uric acid nephropathy (or 'gouty nephropathy') should be thought of as a potential cause of chronic renal failure in a patient with repeated episodes of gout. Renal function is generally mildly impaired and slowly progressive.

PHYSICAL EXAMINATION
Patients with chronic uric acid nephropathy may present with the classical gouty monoarticular arthritis. The affected joint will show signs of

intense inflammation: swelling, erythema, warmth, and exquisite tenderness. Low-grade fever may be present. The skin may show nodular soft tissue prominences in and around the joints (tophi). In advanced cases, joint deformities, secondary to destruction of cartilages and bone are clearly present.

DIFFERENTIAL DIAGNOSIS

In patients presenting with a compatible clinical history, the differential diagnosis of acute uric acid nephropathy should not pose difficulties. On the other hand, the diagnosis of chronic uric acid nephropathy requires that other causes of chronic renal failure are ruled out first. The differential diagnosis includes causes of secondary gout, especially chronic lead nephropathy (saturnine gout). Primary gout is predominantly a male disease, whereas saturnine gout has an equal male:female prevalence. Chronic lead poisoning should be especially suspected in female patients with renal failure and gout. Elevated uric acid levels can also cause renal failure in patients with inherited disorders of purine metabolism (i.e. Lesch–Nyhan syndrome).

INVESTIGATIONS

In acute hyperuricemic nephropathy laboratory abnormalities include hyperkalemia, hyperphosphatemia, hypocalcemia, and acidosis. Urinalysis usually shows massive amounts of uric acid or urate crystals in the sediment. In patients with chronic uric acid nephropathy the diagnosis may be suggested by the presence of hyperuricemia that is disproportional to the degree of renal impairment. Urinalysis is unremarkable except for mild proteinuria.

HISTOLOGY

Acute hyperuricemic nephropathy is characterized by intraluminal precipitation of uric acid crystals, tubular obstruction, and minimal interstitial cellular infiltration. Crystallization is seen predominantly in the medullary collecting ducts.

Chronic uric acid nephropathy is characterized by tubulointerstitial fibrosis. Uric acid crystals (microtophus) can be seen precipitated inside the tubules in the medulla and renal papilla, which gives the appearance of yellow-white nodules or streaks. If tubular disruption occurs, crystals may be seen in the interstitium where they trigger a focal granulomatous interstitial nephritis, consisting of macrophages, multinucleated giant cells, and lymphocytes (111). Ultimately, progressive interstitial fibrosis, arteriolar nephrosclerosis, and glomerulosclerosis develop. Crystals are characteristically needle-shaped and are birefringent under polarized light. Crystalline material can be seen within the tubular lumen of collecting ducts. However, the absence of crystal does not rule out uric acid nephropathy as the initial cause.

PROGNOSIS

With proper prophylaxis, acute nephropathy is rare. For those patients who develop acute renal failure, prognosis is usually good and renal function typically returns to baseline in 7–10 days. Chronic urate nephropathy is a slowly progressive disease.

MANAGEMENT

The best treatment for acute hyperuricemic nephropathy is prevention. Allopurinol, a competitive inhibitor of xanthine oxidase, decreases uric acid production within 48 hours and its use is indicated in patients undergoing chemotherapy. The dose needs to be adjusted for renal function. Forced diuresis helps to maintain a good urine output and reduces tubular concentration of uric acid. In patients developing oliguria, rapid expansion of the extracellular fluid volume and use of diuretics may reverse the acute situation. In addition, urinary alkalinization increases uric acid solubility in the urine. Caution should be taken when alkalinizing the urine when the phosphorus is >7 mg/dl (>2.3 mmol/l) because it can precipitate calcium phosphate crystals and exacerbate intraluminal obstruction. For patients with established acute renal failure, hemodialysis provides an effective clearance of uric acid.

Apart from the general recommendations regarding the management of patients with chronic renal failure, such as treating hypertension, hyperlipidemia, and restriction of protein intake, there is no specific treatment for chronic uric acid nephropathy, except the use of allopurinol to control hyperuricemia.

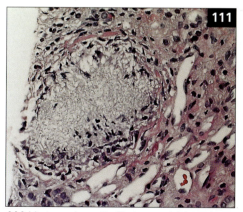

111 Urate nephropathy. Tophus containing uric acid crystals is surrounded by macrophages. Light microscopy (H+E ×400).

Lead nephropathy

DEFINITION
Lead nephropathy is a chronic interstitial nephritis secondary to heavy exposure to lead over a number of years.

EPIDEMIOLOGY AND ETIOLOGY
Certain professions like miners, painters, plumbers, and workers involved in the manufacturing of batteries, pottery and pewter are examples of occupational exposure to lead. Environmental contamination also occurs by ingestion of lead-contaminated food or water. Children under the age of 6 years are at increased risk of lead toxicity in comparison to adults, because of their increased capacity for lead absorption. Other factors that increase the susceptibility to lead toxicity include the amount of calcium and vitamin D in the diet, and iron stores.

PATHOGENESIS
Lead present in the glomerular ultrafiltrate is reabsorbed in the proximal tubule where its accumulation is likely to mediate the pathologic process of lead toxicity, although the precise mechanism is unknown.

CLINICAL HISTORY AND PHYSICAL EXAMINATION
The two main forms of presentation are:
- As part of an acute lead intoxication syndrome, with abdominal pain, hemolytic anemia, peripheral neuropathy, encephalopathy, and proximal tubular dysfunction manifested either as proximal renal tubular acidosis or Fanconi's syndrome, with aminoaciduria, phosphaturia, and glycosuria.
- Chronic lead nephropathy. These patients present similarly to patients with chronic renal failure from other etiologies. Hypertension is usually present. Proteinuria tends to be low (<1g/24 h). Chronic lead toxicity is associated with saturnine gout and renal adenocarcinoma.

DIFFERENTIAL DIAGNOSIS
The main differential diagnosis is with chronic urate nephropathy. A history of occupational lead exposure or presence of urate deposits (tophi) in renal biopsy help in making the correct diagnosis.

INVESTIGATIONS
Urinalysis shows proteinuria, mainly due to low-molecular weight proteins such as β2-microglobulin or retinol-binding protein. Anemia is characterized by the presence of 'basophilic stippling'. Hyperuricemia is secondary to reduced urate secretion by the impaired proximal tubules. In adults, the best screening tests for lead exposure are lead levels in the blood and erythrocyte protoporphyrin. In children, where significant lead toxicity can occur with low-level exposure, measurement of blood lead levels is the primary screening method. In addition, determination of urinary lead excretion after administration of a lead chelator such as calcium disodium salt of ethylene diamine tetra-acetic acid (EDTA) can be used to document excessive lead absorption in patients with chronic low levels of lead exposure.

HISTOLOGY
In acute lead nephropathy renal biopsy shows proximal tubular injury, with intranuclear inclusion bodies composed of a lead–protein complex. With chronic lead nephropathy kidneys are shrunken (**112**). On histology there is a nonspecific interstitial nephritis and tubular atrophy that is indistinguishable from other forms of nephrosclerosis.

PROGNOSIS
In patients in whom the main manifestation of lead nephrotoxicity is abnormal proximal tubular function, prognosis is good and usually reversible. Chronic lead nephropathy is considered to be irreversible, with patients slowly progressing to end-stage renal disease.

MANAGEMENT
Preventive measures, such removal of lead from gasoline and paint, have reduced the risk of lead toxicity in the general population. Initial treatment involves removal of the source of lead. Blood lead levels ≥45 µg/dl (2.2 µmol/l) in children, and ≥70 µg/dl (3.4 µmol/l) in adults, are an indication for chelation therapy.

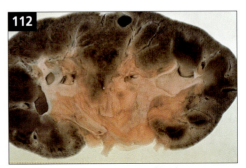

112 Macroscopic appearance of lead nephropathy. The kidney is small secondary to cortical loss and has a smooth outer surface.

Lithium-induced renal disease

DEFINITION
Lithium is an effective drug in the control of bipolar affective disorders. However long-term use is frequently complicated by nephrotoxicity.

EPIDEMIOLOGY
Patients with severe unipolar and bipolar affective disorders are at increased risk of lithium toxicity.

PATHOGENESIS
Lithium is freely filtered at the glomerulus with re-absorption occurring at several places along the nephron. In the renal medulla, lithium transport into the collecting tubule cells occurs via sodium channels in the luminal membrane. In this nephron segment, lithium accumulation interferes with the ability of vasopressin to increase water re-absorption by at least two mechanisms:
- Direct inhibition of the adenylate cyclase system.
- Inhibition of transepithelial water movement by down-regulating the expression of aquaporin 2.

CLINICAL HISTORY AND PHYSICAL EXAMINATION
The renal manifestations of lithium toxicity include:
- Nephrogenic diabetes insipidus.
- Type 1 (distal) renal tubular acidosis (RTA).
- Nephrotic syndrome.
- Acute tubular necrosis (ATN).
- Chronic interstitial nephritis.

Nephrogenic diabetes is suggested by the presence of polyuria and polydipsia in up to 40% of patients. RTA is incomplete and rarely of clinical significance. Nephrotic syndrome is secondary to minimal change nephropathy and remits upon lithium withdrawal. ATN may be the presenting feature following acute lithium intoxication. In patients with lithium-induced chronic interstitial nephritis, GFR is usually modestly reduced. Physical examination is unrevealing.

DIFFERENTIAL DIAGNOSIS
The differential diagnosis includes other causes of polyuria and mild renal failure such as diabetes mellitus, chronic interstitial nephritis, and Fanconi syndrome.

INVESTIGATIONS
Investigations include a determination of lithium levels and estimation of the glomerular filtration rate and of the 24-hour urine volume. In patients with elevated creatinine a renal biopsy should be considered.

HISTOLOGY
Lithium-induced ATN is characterized by cell ballooning, swelling, and vacuolation mostly seen in the distal convoluted tubules. In patients with chronic lithium nephropathy biopsies show a focal chronic interstitial nephropathy, with interstitial fibrosis, tubular atrophy, and glomerular sclerosis (**113**). Characteristically there is cystic dilatation of the distal tubules.

PROGNOSIS
Nephrogenic diabetes insipidus is usually reversible once lithium intake has been discontinued, although in some cases abnormaliies in urinary concentration may persist for many months. Patients with a clinical history complicated by repeated episodes of lithium intoxication may show a sustained increase in serum creatinine. However, the role of lithium in causing end-stage renal failure is controversial.

MANAGEMENT
For patients with mild lithium intoxication, treatment of acute lithium intoxication includes admitting the patient to the hospital, discontinuation of the drug, and vigorous restoration of extracellular volume depletion. For patients with severe lithium intoxication, hemodialysis is the treatment of choice. Lithium levels may rebound following dialysis. Thiazide diuretics should be avoided in patients on lithium therapy because the volume contraction can result in an increase in proximal tubule reabsorption of sodium and lithium that together can precipitate an episode of acute lithium intoxication. Patient on long-term lithium therapy should have their renal function checked at least once a year. Lithium therapy should be discontinued if there is evidence of progressive renal function decline.

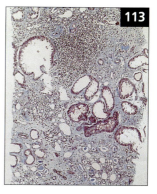

113 Lithium-induced renal disease. Extensive interstitial fibrosis and tubular atrophy is seen with a chronic lymphocytic inflammatory infiltrate. Light microscopy (H+E ×100).

Radiation nephritis

DEFINITION

Radiation nephritis is an inflammatory, thrombotic and degenerative disorder of the kidney that is secondary to the effects of ionizing radiation.

EPIDEMIOLOGY

In general, direct exposure of >50% of the kidney to 20–30 Gy (2000–3000 rad) during a period of 5 weeks or less will result in nephritis. Minimizing the total dose of irradiation to <20–30 Gy (2000–3000 rads), proper shielding of the kidneys, and/or fractionation of the total body irradiation into several small doses over several days has resulted in the virtual disappearance of radiation nephritis.

PATHOGENESIS

In experimental models, direct irradiation of the kidney results in degeneration of the glomerular tuft and tubular epithelial cells, associated with inflammatory interstitial infiltrates. With time, there is progressive glomerular sclerosis, tubular atrophy, and interstitial fibrosis. Renal endothelial cells appear to be the initial target of ionizing radiation. There is a suggestion that endothelial cell injury may be mediated by the generation of oxygen free radicals, formed by radiation-induced enzyme activation. The sensitivity of the endothelial cells to radiation is increased by some antineoplastic medications. Increased sensitivity of the kidney to radiation has been noted with use of actinomycin-D, bleomycin, vinblastine, and cyclophosphamide.

CLINICAL HISTORY AND PHYSICAL EXAMINATION

There are four clinical syndromes associated with renal irradiation in excess of 20 Gy (2000 rads):

- Acute radiation nephritis: occurs in 40% of patients after a latency of 6–12 months. Patients typically present with abrupt onset of hypertension, proteinuria, edema, and progressive renal failure.
- Chronic radiation nephritis: usually manifested by insidious onset of hypertension and proteinuria that develops in a patient ≥1 year after irradiation. There is gradual loss of renal function.
- Benign hypertension: may occur ≥2 years after exposure to radiation. Hypertension is associated with variable proteinuria and normal renal function, a good long-term prognosis.
- Malignant hypertension: can present months to years after radiation. Patients in this group have a poor prognosis.

DIFFERENTIAL DIAGNOSIS

Because of morphologic similarities, the main differential diagnoses are hemolytic uremic syndrome and thrombocytopenic purpura.

INVESTIGATIONS

Laboratory abnormalities include proteinuria (may be nephrotic), little or no hematuria, anemia, and elevated creatinine.

HISTOLOGY

Histologic features may vary, depending on the dose of radiation administered and the time of the biopsy. In mild cases, glomeruli show mesangial cell proliferation and matrix expansion, with occasional areas of mesangiolysis. Typically the capillary walls appear thickened and show 'splitting'. In severe cases, glomeruli may show fibrinoid necrosis and thrombosis, and epithelial crescents are not unusual. Larger vessels may be normal or show patchy intimal proliferation with increased thickness, intimal fibrosis, or fibrinoid necrosis (**114**). The interstitium may show interstitial infiltrates, tubular atrophy, and interstitial fibrosis. Interstitial changes may occur in the absence of glomerular abnormalities. On immunofluorescence, immunoglobulins and fibrin may be seen deposited along the capillary walls. Electron microscopy shows splitting of the capillary wall due to interposition of mesangial matrix between the glomerular basement membrane and the endothelial cells. The subendothelial space is widened by deposition of a nondescript amorphous material.

PROGNOSIS

Acute radiation nephritis may resolve spontaneously in some cases. More frequently, it progresses to chronic radiation nephritis. Malignant hypertension and impaired renal function early on presentation indicate a poor prognosis.

MANAGEMENT

Treatment is supportive, with care taken to control blood pressure and risk factors for renal disease progression. In experimental models, ACE inhibitors have been shown to reduce the progression of renal disease and improve survival. As in many other conditions, the best treatment is prevention. The risk of developing radiation nephritis may be reduced by keeping the total dose of radiation to the kidney to <20–30 Gy (2000–3000 rads), fractionating the total dose into several small doses over several days, and proper shielding of the kidneys.

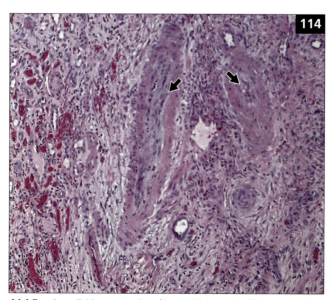

114 Focal medial hypertrophy of interstitial arteries. These vessels (arrows) show endothelial cell swelling, subintimal deposition of basophilic material, severe interstitial fibrosis, and tubular atrophy. Light microscopy (H+E ×200).

Chapter Five

Diseases affecting the renal vasculature

- **Atheromatous renovascular disease**

- **Fibromuscular renovascular disease**

- **Cholesterol emboli**

- **Essential hypertension and the kidney**

- **Scleroderma**

- **Hemolytic–uremic syndrome (HUS)**

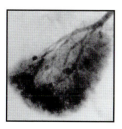
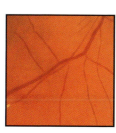
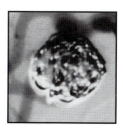
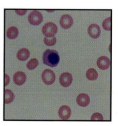

Atheromatous renovascular disease

DEFINITION
Atheroma of the renal arteries can cause stenosis or occlusion of the vessels leading to hypertension or renal impairment. It is the commonest cause of renovascular disease. Atherosclerotic lesions of the renal artery typically occur in the ostium or proximal renal artery and are eccentric rather than concentric in nature. Lesions are commonly bilateral. The natural history is of progressive narrowing of the stenosis leading eventually to occlusion.

EPIDEMIOLOGY AND ETIOLOGY
Atheromatous renovascular disease is extremely common in patients who have evidence of generalized atherosclerosis. If hypertensive patients with coronary artery disease or peripheral vascular disease are screened by renal angiography, 30–50% will be found to have a renal artery stenosis. Advanced age, diabetes mellitus, hypertension, hypercholesterolemia, and smoking are risk factors. It is a common cause of end-stage renal failure in the elderly population.

PATHOGENESIS
If a unilateral stenosis is severe there may be tubular atrophy and interstitial fibrosis on the side ipsilateral to the stenosis due to long-standing ischemia, and possibly cholesterol embolization. The ischemic kidney secretes renin which leads to increased angiotensin II production. The resultant hypertension may in time cause nephrosclerosis in the contralateral kidney.

CLINICAL HISTORY
Patients with atheromatous renovasular disease usually present with hypertension and/or renal impairment. Sometimes the deterioration in renal function follows commencement of an ACE inhibitor. Another classic presentation is with recurrent pulmonary edema, usually in patients with bilateral disease. Proteinuria is common and occasionally may be in the nephrotic range.

PHYSICAL EXAMINATION
Renal artery bruits may be audible. There is commonly evidence of generalized atherosclerosis, e.g. absent foot pulses, carotid artery bruits.

DIFFERENTIAL DIAGNOSIS
Although atheroma is the commonest cause of renal artery stenosis, other conditions can cause it. The commonest is fibromuscular dysplasia. In children, coarctation of the aorta or narrowing of the aorta in association with neurofibromatosis are important causes (**115**). Large or medium vessel vasculitides such as polyarteritis nodosa, giant cell arteritis, syphilis, and Takayasu's arteritis can cause renal artery stenosis (**116**). Renal or adrenal tumors or even large simple renal cysts may compress the renal artery, producing hypertension.

INVESTIGATIONS
Ultrasound is a useful initial imaging technique because the presence of asymmetric kidneys in a patient with other evidence of vascular disease is very suggestive of renal arterial disease. Renal angiography (**117**) is the gold standard investigation but is invasive and the dye is potentially nephrotoxic. Pressure gradients can be measured at the time of angiography if it is not certain from the images obtained whether the stenosis is critical. Various noninvasive tests can be of use. Captopril-DTPA scans can be useful functional tests of the significance of a renal artery stenosis. The functionality of a significant unilateral renal artery stenosis is demonstrated by a fall in the single kidney GFR after ACE I administration, relative to that of the contralateral kidney (**118, 119**). Duplex Doppler ultrasound is not a reliable screening investigation in most centers. Magnetic resonance angiography (MRA) is becoming a reliable noninvasive alternative to conventional angiography. It does not require arterial catheterization or administration of nephrotoxic drugs (**120, 121**).

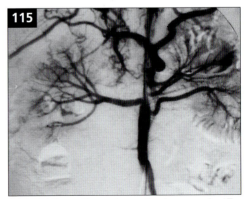

115

115 Middle aortic syndrome. Aortogram of a 17-year-old male with severe hypertension showing typical feature of the middle aortic syndrome. Note the severe tubular stenosis involving most of the abdominal aorta. There are multiple renal arteries that are stenosed. The superior mesenteric artery is also severely stenosed.

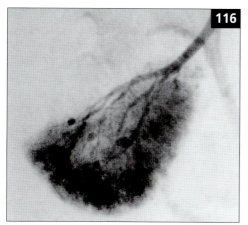

116 Polyarteritis nodosa. A selective injection of a lower pole branch artery shows typical microaneurysms.

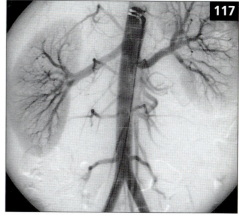

117 Intra-arterial digital subtraction angiogram (DSA) showing normal renal arteries.

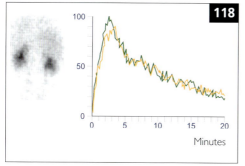

118 Precaptopril renogram in a patient with bilateral renal artery stenosis. Transit time: right kidney 198 s, left kidney 177 s.

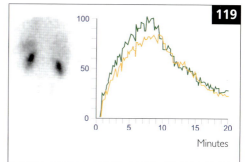

119 Postcaptopril renogram showing delayed transit times bilaterally. Transit time: right kidney 398 s, left kidney 377 s.

120 Magnetic resonance angiogram showing total occlusion of the right renal artery and stenosis of the proximal left renal artery.

121 Corresponding DSA.

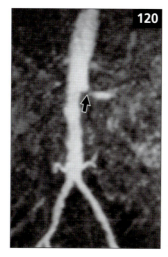

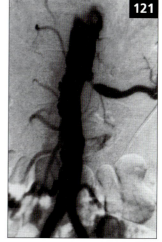

Atheromatous renovascular disease (*continued*)

Renal artery occlusion may occur spontaneously due to thrombosis or embolism (**122**) or as a result of trauma. Trauma can cause renal artery occlusion by raising an intimal flap or causing a dissection of the renal artery (**123**). Causes of traumatic renal artery thrombosis include blunt trauma, or iatrogenic trauma complicating such procedures as nephrolithotomy, nephrostomy, renal biopsy or, most commonly, percutaneous transluminal renal angioplasty (PTRA). Acute renal artery occlusion in a previously normal artery leads rapidly to infarction presenting as loin pain, fever, and vomiting. Thrombosis of a solitary kidney or bilateral renal artery thrombosis will cause anuric acute renal failure. More commonly thrombosis is superimposed on a pre-existing progressive renal artery stenosis. The ischemic kidney will have developed an extensive collateral circulation from intercostal, lumbar, adrenal, gonadal, and ureteric vessels. As a result infarction does not occur and the occlusion is usually asymptomatic, although there may be worsening of hypertension and renal function.

Renal artery aneurysms (**124, 125**) are usually due to atherosclerosis but can be caused by any of the above mentioned diseases. Complications include rupture, thrombosis, hypertension, distal embolization, and formation of an arteriovenous fistula.

PROGNOSIS

Atheromatous renovascular disease is progressive so stenoses tend to become more critical and eventually occlude. It is also common for the disease to become bilateral over time. Renovascular disease is part of a generalized process and patients often die from coronary or cerebrovascular disease before they develop end-stage renal failure.

MANAGEMENT

Medical management consists of optimizing blood pressure control, and lowering serum cholesterol levels. The role of PTRA and surgery remains controversial. Most centers will use PTRA rather than surgery as it is much less invasive in often elderly high-risk patients. Stenting

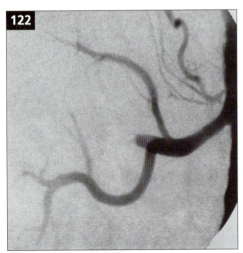

122 Renal artery embolism. On an earlier aortogram the whole of the right renal artery was demonstrated. On this subsequent study the middle branch is occluded with a sharp cut-off. These appearances are typical of embolism.

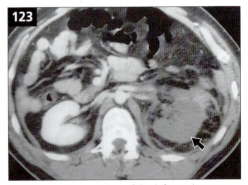

123 Traumatic occlusion of the left renal artery following a road traffic accident. On enhanced CT note the absence of contrast medium in the left renal artery and the lack of enhancement of the kidney (arrow).

is now often performed following angioplasty. PTRA has been shown to improve blood pressure control in a proportion of patients but its effect on renal function may be to worsen or improve it.

Patients most likely to benefit from PTRA are those with very severe stenoses, rapid deterioration in renal function and a >9 cm (3.5 in) in length kidney beyond the stenosis (**126, 127**). Surgery is indicated in patients unsuitable for PTRA, where the aorta needs to be reconstructed, and in patients with an occluded renal artery but evidence of good collateral blood flow and evidence of a viable kidney.

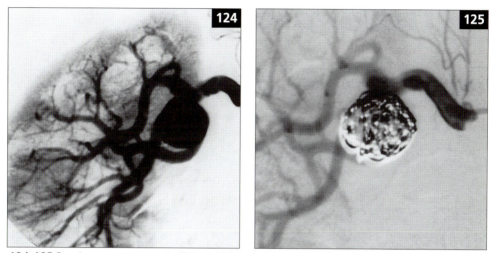

124, 125 Renal artery aneurysm. A 60-yearold female presented with severe hypertension. An aneurysm measuring 3 cm (1.2 in) in diameter is demonstrated at the renal hilum with a relatively narrow neck (**124**). It was possible to place coils safely within the aneurysm. The final postembolization procedure shows that the arterial supply to the kidney is unaffected (**125**).

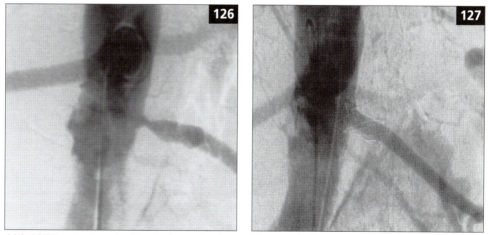

126, 127 Renal artery stenting. Aortography shows diffuse aortic disease with an occluded right renal artery and a severe proximal stenosis on the left (**126**). Primary stenting was performed. A follow-up study 27 months later demonstrates a satisfactory angiographic appearance with the stent just protruding into the aorta (**127**).

Fibromuscular renovascular disease

DEFINITION
Fibromuscular disease typically affects the middle or distal portions of the renal arteries. It may affect other vessels most commonly the carotid arteries, but also the subclavian, coronary, mesenteric, and iliac arteries. Most commonly it affects the medial muscular layer with medial fibroplasia in 85% and medial hyperplasia in 10%. Typically lesions are multiple and stenotic segments are linked by aneurysmal areas, giving a strings-of-beads appearance on angiography.

EPIDEMIOLOGY AND ETIOLOGY
Fibromuscular disease is the commonest form of renovascular disease in young adults. It is about six times more common in females than males. It is rare in blacks.

PATHOGENESIS
The pathogenesis of fibromuscular dysplasia is unknown.

CLINICAL HISTORY AND PHYSICAL EXAMINATION
Fibromuscular disease should be considered in patients, typically females, who present with hypertension before the age of 25 years in the absence of a strong family history of essential hypertension.

INVESTIGATIONS
Diagnosis is made by renal angiography (**128**).

PROGNOSIS
The natural history of untreated fibromuscular dysplasia is not well-described, especially as most cases are now treated by PTRA. A proportion of cases can progress to occlusion.

MANAGEMENT
PTRA is more successful in patients with fibromuscular disease than atheromatous renovascular disease at curing or improving hypertension. Re-stenosis is also less likely. PTRA is thus the treatment of choice, allowing the patient a chance of discontinuing antihypertensive medication.

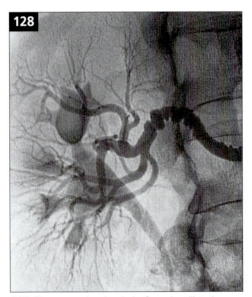

128 Fibromuscular dysplasia. Saccular dilatations and web-like stenoses are seen affecting the distal right renal artery.

Cholesterol emboli

DEFINITION
Cholesterol crystals that embolize to the renal circulation lodge in the small arteries or afferent arterioles and set up an inflammatory reaction which compromises renal function.

EPIDEMIOLOGY AND ETIOLOGY
Cholesterol embolization occurs in elderly patients with generalized atherosclerosis. It may occur spontaneously from ruptured aortic atheromatous plaques but more commonly occurs after interventional procedures which dislodge cholesterol from the aortic wall, or after anticoagulation or thrombolysis which lead to hemorrhage into a plaque with subsequent dislodgement of cholesterol crystals. Cholesterol emboli may also be found downstream of a significant renal artery stenosis.

PATHOGENESIS
Cholesterol crystals cause vascular occlusion and incite a foreign body giant cell reaction with a mononuclear cell infiltrate which leads to interstitial fibrosis, tubular atrophy, and intravascular fibrosis.

CLINICAL HISTORY
Patients may present with oliguric acute renal failure or slowly progressive renal insufficiency. Microscopic hematuria and minor proteinuria may be present. Patients often have symptoms of other organ involvement if cholesterol emboli have showered into other circulations. There may be an acute confusional state or focal neurologic deficits, pancreatitis, or gastrointestinal bleeding.

PHYSICAL EXAMINATION
Common findings are livedo reticularis and gangrene of the toes, often with normal pedal pulses (trash feet). Fundoscopy may show emboli lodged at branch points in the retinal arterioles (Hollenhorst plaques) (**129**).

INVESTIGATIONS
Typically the ESR is raised, there is eosinophilia and serum complement levels are depressed.

HISTOLOGY
Sites of emboli are recognized by cleft or needle-like spaces usually within the interlobular and arcuate vessels (**130**), but may also be seen in glomerular capillaries. The presence of cholesterol rapidly incites a foreign body giant cell reaction. The vessels will usually show intimal thickening and fibrosis. Rarely, a crescentic glomerulonephritis can occur.

PROGNOSIS
The outcome for these patients is generally poor and is determined by the severity of the vascular disease and degree of embolization that has occurred. Renal function usually declines progressively.

MANAGEMENT
Interventional vascular procedures and anti-coagulation are contra-indicated. There have been reports of renal function stabilizing in patients treated aggressively with statins to lower the serum cholesterol levels.

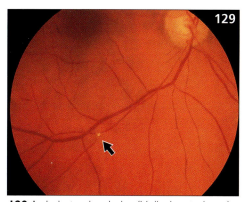

129 A cholesterol embolus (Hollenhorst plaque) (arrow) can be seen lodged at the bifurcation of the inferior branch retinal artery.

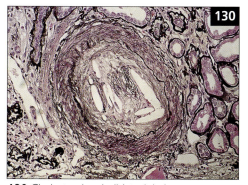

130 Cholesterol emboli. Interlobular artery shows complete occlusion with large cholesterol clefts. Light microscopy (MS ×250).

Essential hypertension and the kidney

DEFINITION
Renal function and blood pressure are intimately linked: primary renal disease causes hypertension, and hypertension impairs renal function. In the absence of primary renal disease, essential hypertension can cause structural changes in the kidney which are at their most florid in accelerated hypertension.

EPIDEMIOLOGY AND ETIOLOGY
In whites it is debated whether essential hypertension, without an accelerated phase, can cause end-stage renal failure. In the European Dialysis and Transplantation Association Registry in 1986, hypertension was documented as the cause of renal failure in 6.1% of patients. Blacks seem to be much more likely to develop renal failure as a consequence of hypertension.

PATHOGENESIS
The morphologic effects of hypertension on the kidney can be studied in the Goldblatt rat model of two-kidney, one-clip hypertension, by examining renal histology in the kidney contralateral to the renal clip. The changes seen in the kidney are similar to those seen in humans with essential hypertension. The initial change is medial hypertrophy of the intrarenal arterial and arteriolar wall, followed by segmental hyalinosis of the vessel wall, probably due to breakdown of autoregulation and intrusion of blood vessel constituents into the vessel wall. At a later stage focal and segmental glomerulosclerosis with tubular atrophy develops. The final stage involves severe concentric intimal fibrosis of the interlobular arteries. If the clip is removed after one year, the blood pressure decreases temporarily and then, after 1 week, returns to the hypertensive levels. Normotension is regained if the previously untouched kidney is removed, indicating the importance of the hypertension-induced structural changes in maintaining the hypertensive state.

CLINICAL HISTORY
Usually hypertension is asymptomatic until it reaches the accelerated phase.

Then patients may complain of headache, visual disturbance, or symptoms of heart failure. In accelerated hypertension proteinuria is commonly present, and may reach nephrotic range, and largely resolves after treatment of the hypertension.

PHYSICAL EXAMINATION
Patients with essential hypertension may have clinical signs of left ventricular hypertension. Accelerated hypertension causes loss of autoregulation in the retinal vessels leading to hard exudates formed by constituents of plasma and hemorrhage (**131**). Soft exudates (cotton wool spots) are caused by ischemic infarction of nerve fibers. Papilloedema is a swelling of the optic disk with loss of the disk margins.

INVESTIGATIONS
Essential hypertension over time leads to left ventricular hypertrophy which is seen on echocardiography. Accelerated hypertension leads to elevated renin and aldosterone levels which lead to a hypokalemic metabolic alkalosis.

HISTOLOGY
The effects of essential hypertension in stable phase on the kidney have traditionally been termed nephrosclerosis. There is segmental hyalinization of interlobular arteries and afferent arterioles, which leads to ischemic collapse of the glomerular tuft and focal glomerulosclerosis. There will then be atrophy of the tubules related to that glomerulus (individual nephron damage). This will eventually lead on to cortical atrophy and renal failure. In accelerated hypertension there is a proliferative intimal arteritis of the interlobular arteries, leading to almost complete occlusion of the lumen with the so-called onion skin lesion (**132, 133**). There is also fibrinoid necrosis of the afferent arterioles which may extend into the glomerular tuft to cause focal and segmental necrosis, sometimes with crescent formation.

PROGNOSIS
Patients with accelerated hypertension and acute renal failure with no pre-existing renal disease will often recover significant renal function after blood pressure is brought under control.

MANAGEMENT
Optimal control of essential hypertension is important to prevent the development of atherosclerosis leading especially to coronary and cerebrovascular disease.

131 Superficial and deep retinal hemorrhages are seen in a patient with accelerated hypertension. There is comparatively little change in the retinal arteries themselves, indicating that the hypertension is of relatively acute onset.

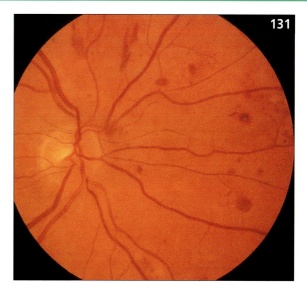

132 Essential hypertension. Large interlobular artery showing extensive reduplication of the internal elastic lamina. Light microscopy (MS x250).

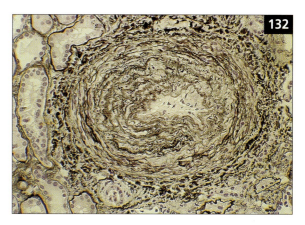

133 Accelerated hypertension. Small interlobular artery is shown in which there is onion skin proliferation (arrow) and fibrinoid necrosis (arrow head) of the arteriole at the hilum. Light microscopy (MS x250).

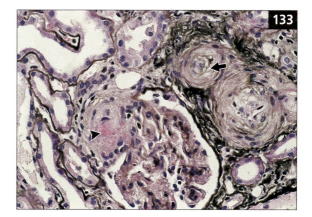

Scleroderma

DEFINITION

Scleroderma is a disease characterized by progressive and irreversible accumulation of connective tissue in the skin and often in visceral organs, together with structural changes in the microvasculature. The disease varies in severity and extent from patches of hard skin (morphoea) to life-threatening systemic illness. Generalized scleroderma can be divided into three subgroups.

Subgroup one:
- Diffuse cutaneous systemic sclerosis.
- Onset of Raynaud's phenomenon within 1 year of onset of skin changes.
- Truncal and acral skin involvement.
- Early and severe incidence of interstitial lung disease, renal failure, gastrointestinal disease, and myocardial disease.
- Absence of anti-centromere antibodies.

Subgroup two:
- Limited cutaneous systemic sclerosis (CREST syndrome).
- Isolated Raynaud's phenomenon for years.
- Scleroderma limited to hands and feet.
- Late incidence of pulmonary hypertension, skin calcinosis, and telangiectasia.
- High incidence of anti-centromere antibodies.

Subgroup three:
- Scleroderma sine scleroderma.
- Visceral disease without cutaneous involvement.

EPIDEMIOLOGY

In the US the incidence is about 10 new cases/million/year. The average age of onset is 30–50 years, and is much more common in females. There is an association with HLA DR3, DR5 and C4 null alleles.

ETIOLOGY AND PATHOGENESIS

The etiology of scleroderma is poorly understood. One interesting hypothesis is that in some women it may be triggered by fetal cells causing a graft versus host type disease. Whatever initiates the process there is overactivity of fibroblasts and endothelial cells leading to increased production of connective tissue. Scleroderma renal crisis is probably caused when a Raynaud's type renal vasoconstriction is superimposed on more chronic structural changes to the vessels.

CLINICAL HISTORY

Renal disease may present with hypertension, proteinuria, and slowly progressive renal impairment. Scleroderma renal crisis tends to occur in patients with rapidly progressive and diffuse cutaneous systemic sclerosis. Patients usually have accelerated hypertension often with headaches, confusion, and visual impairment, and become oligoanuric rapidly. Scleroderma renal crisis can be triggered by cold weather, pregnancy, or by corticosteroids.

PHYSICAL EXAMINATION

Patients with scleroderma renal crisis may have signs of accelerated hypertension. They usually exhibit Raynaud's phenomenon and diffuse scleroderma (**134, 135**).

INVESTIGATIONS

Renal size on ultrasound is usually normal. In diffuse cutaneous systemic sclerosis anti-centromere antibodies are usually absent. Anti-Scl 70 antibodies are found in 30–60% of cases.

HISTOLOGY

The earliest changes in the arcuate and interlobular arteries are of intimal proliferation and edema, followed by perivascular fibrosis. There may be fibrinoid necrosis affecting the small arteries and arterioles indistinguishable from the changes of acclerated hypertension. The glomerular changes are secondary to ischemia.

PROGNOSIS

Scleroderma renal crisis, untreated, will lead to end-stage renal failure and death from accelerated hypertension. However, treatment with ACE inhibitors can lead to recovery of renal function even after dialysis has been initiated.

MANAGEMENT

Avoidance of cold and calcium channel blockers is useful for managing Raynaud's phenomenon. Patients with diffuse cutaneous systemic sclerosis should have their blood pressure and creatinine clearance measured regularly for any sign of deterioration. Various immunosuppressive agents have been tried and much current interest is focussed on mycophenolate mofetil and sirolimus.

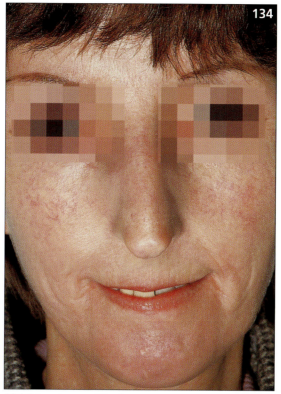

134 Scleroderma of the face.

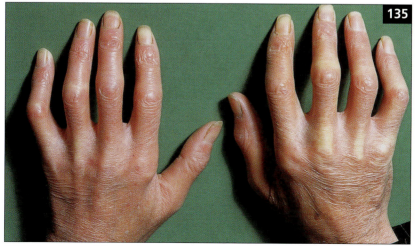

135 Scleroderma of the hands.

Hemolytic–uremic syndrome (HUS)

DEFINITION

Most patients with HUS have different clinical features from patients with thrombotic thrombocytopenic purpura (TTP), although some patients may be difficult to differentiate. Both conditions cause a microangiopathic hemolytic anemia and thrombocytopenia, with HUS more commonly causing renal failure and TTP neurologic symptoms. HUS is classified into typical diarrhea associated D+, or atypical D- forms.

EPIDEMIOLOGY AND ETIOLOGY

D+ HUS occurs mainly in young children, but can occur in adults. It is usually caused by ingestion of meat containing *E. coli* 0157:H7. This produces shiga-like toxins which bind to a glycolipid receptor, galactotriosylceramide (Gb3) on renal endothelial cells, and trigger endothelial damage. D- HUS may be inherited or associated with *Streptococcus pneumoniae* infection, HIV, pregnancy, oral contraceptives, systemic lupus erythematosus especially with anti-phospholipid antibodies, cyclosporine (cyclosporin) and tacrolimus, mucin-secreting carcinoma, and mitomycin-C. TTP is now thought to be due either to a genetic deficency of von Willebrand factor converting enzyme or to auto-antibody production directed against this enzyme, possibly triggered by infection.

PATHOGENESIS

Endothelial injury leads to a prothrombotic state by a variety of mechanisms, including reduced prostacyclin and nitric oxide production and increased release of von Willebrand factor multimers by endothelial cells.

CLINICAL HISTORY AND PHYSICAL EXAMINATION

D+ HUS often occurs after bloody diarrhea has started to improve. It presents as weakness, pallor, and purpura. Oligoanuria may develop together with hypertension and signs of fluid overload. Uremia and hyponatremia may cause neurologic symptoms such as confusion and seizures.

INVESTIGATIONS

Thrombocytopenia and hemolytic anemia are found. Fragmented red blood cells, schistocytes, are found in the peripheral blood film (**136**). Markers of hemolysis include elevated lactate dehyrogenase (LDH), unconjugated bilirubin levels and reticulocyte levels, and low haptoglobin levels.

HISTOLOGY

HUS/TTP cause thrombosis of intrarenal vessels in the absence of cellular inflammation. In D+ HUS there is mainly glomerular capillary thrombosis, whereas in other forms there is predominant involvement of the small arteries with a florid intimal mucoid proliferation of arteries and arterioles with onion-skinning and thrombosis (**137–139**). Acute tubular necrosis occurs in proportion to the vascular pathology. Immunohistochemistry shows fibrin in areas of thrombus formation, but no immunoglobulin deposition. Electron microscopy shows a characteristic area of electron lucency between the basement membrane and the swollen endothelium (**140**).

PROGNOSIS

D+ HUS has a current mortality of 6%, and complete recovery of renal function normally occurs within 2 or 3 weeks. In adults with HUS, prognosis is worse. Older age is associated with increased mortality in the acute phase, whereas severe renal involvement at the onset of disease is associated with an unfavorable long-term renal prognosis.

MANAGEMENT

Anemia is managed by blood transfusion and renal failure by dialysis if necessary. D+ HUS does not respond to FFP or plasma exchange, whereas D- HUS should be managed by treating any underlying disease and with plasma exchange. Platelet transfusions should be avoided unless there is active bleeding, because there is a risk of accelerating the process. Familial HUS recurs commonly after renal transplantation.

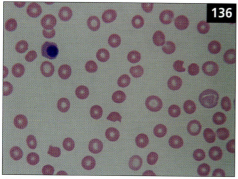

136 Blood film showing fragmented red cells (under oil immersion x500).

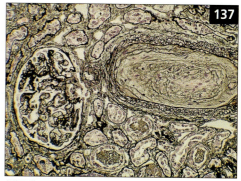

137 Occlusive mucoid intimal proliferation in an interlobular artery. Light microscopy (MS x250).

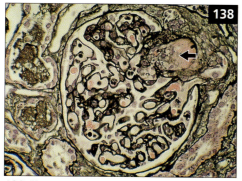

138 Glomerulus showing arteriolar thrombus (arrow). Light microscopy (MS x400).

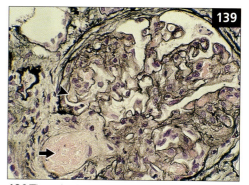

139 Thrombotic thrombocytopenic purpura. Glomerulus showing arteriolar (arrow) and capillary tuft thrombus (arrow head). Light microscopy (MS x400).

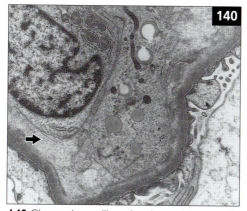

140 Glomerular capillary showing a wide area of subendothelial lucency (arrow). Electron microscopy (x5000).

Chapter Six

Renal infections and structural abnormalities

- **Acute pyelonephritis**

- **Xanthogranulomatous pyelonephritis**

- **Malakoplakia**

- **Renal tuberculosis**

- **Two unusual renal infections**

- **Vesicoureteric reflux and reflux nephropathy**

- **Urinary tract obstruction**

- **Congenital anomalies of the urinary tract**

- **Renal calculi**

- **Retroperitoneal fibrosis**

- **Medullary sponge kidney**

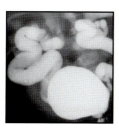
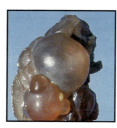
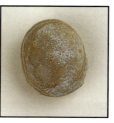
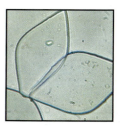

Acute pyelonephritis

DEFINITION
Acute pyelonephritis is an infection of the renal parenchyma usually by bacteria which have ascended the urinary tract. Renal abscesses are usually caused by hematogenous spread to the kidney.

EPIDEMIOLOGY AND ETIOLOGY
Acute pyelonephritis, like acute cystitis, is much more common in females than in males. Risk factors include sexual intercourse, instrumentation of the urinary tract, structural abnormalities of the urinary tract including obstruction and vesicoureteric reflux, pregnancy, diabetes mellitus, and asymptomatic bacteriuria. Urinary tract infections usually occur in males aged over 40 years and are often associated with prostatic disease or urinary tract calculi. The most common pathogens are organisms that are normal bowel flora, *Escherichia coli, Proteus, Pseudomonas* and *Klebsiella* species. Approximately 10–15% of infections are due to Gram-positive organisms, mainly staphylococcal species and *Enterococcus fecalis.*

PATHOGENESIS
The first step is colonization of the lower vagina and periurethral area with uropathogenic bacteria originating from the gut flora, followed by transurethral passage of the bacteria and bladder infection. Whether bacteria ascend the urinary tract to cause acute pyelonephritis is due to a poorly-understood interplay between host defences and bacterial virulence. The renal medulla is the first area of renal parenchyma to be infected.

CLINICAL HISTORY AND PHYSICAL EXAMINATION
Patients usually present with high fever, rigors, loin pain and usually lower tract symptoms of dysuria, urgency, and frequency. Bacteremia and septic shock may develop, usually in association with obstruction or immunosuppression.

DIFFERENTIAL DIAGNOSIS
The symptoms and signs of acute pyelonephritis may be mimicked by obstructive uropathy, acute glomerulonephritis, renal infarction, pneumonia, acute pancreatitis, and other intra-abdominal conditions.

INVESTIGATIONS
Urine microscopy reveals pyuria (more than five white blood cells/high-powered field) and bacteriuria (one or more bacterium per oil immersion field on a Gram-stained field of uncentrifuged urine), and the presence of white blood cell or bacterial casts confirms renal parenchymal invasion (**141**). Urinalysis sticks detect white cells by measuring leucocyte esterase, and bacteriuria by the demonstration of nitrites produced by the bacterial reduction of nitrate normally present in urine. Blood and urine cultures must be performed. Significant bacteriuria is conventionally defined as the presence of 10^5 or more of the same organism per ml. However, many patients are symptomatic with lower bacterial counts.

Ultrasound shows renal enlargement and is mainly useful at excluding obstruction. Intravenous urography is indicated after acute pyelonephritis has been treated if the episode has been severe, slow to resolve, or relapsing. It provides excellent imaging of the calyces, pelvis, and ureter. Intravenous urography is good at detecting obstruction, stones, papillary necrosis, or stones.

In severe cases there may be a solid inflammatory mass without drainable pus, termed acute focal bacterial pyelonephritis, which can progress to intrarenal and perirenal abscess formation which is best imaged by CT.

Emphysematous pyelonephritis is a rare form of acute pyelonephritis, found most often in diabetics and alcoholics, that is best imaged by CT (**142**).

HISTOLOGY
Renal biopsy is rarely indicated in acute pyelonephritis. Histologic appearances are of pus-filled abscesses within the cortex and medulla. If associated with an ascending infection, pus will be seen radiating up from the pelvis within collecting ducts and tubules.

PROGNOSIS
Acute pyelonephritis in patients with normal upper tracts is usually easily treated and leaves no permanent structural or functional damage. Renal infection associated with obstruction or stones may lead to irreversible renal damage.

MANAGEMENT
Parenteral antibiotics are needed for patients with obstruction or stones, and in older patients in whom sepsis is more common. Obstruction must be dealt with as a medical emergency. Oral antibiotics can be given to younger patients who have no evidence of systemic sepsis and no complicating factors.

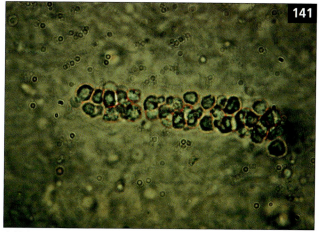

141 Urine microscopy demonstrating a white cell cast.

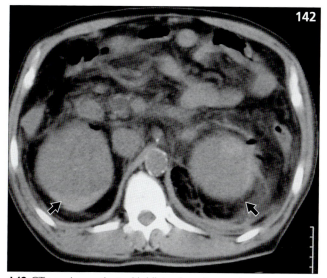

142 CT scan in a patient with bilateral emphysematous pyelonephritis demonstrating grossly enlarged kidneys with air within the parenchyma (arrows).

Xanthogranulomatous pyelonephritis

DEFINITION
Xanthogranulomatous pyelonephritis is characterized by chronic granulomatous infiltration of the kidney with prominent collections of foam cells.

EPIDEMIOLOGY AND ETIOLOGY
It mainly affects females and is most common in the elderly.

PATHOGENESIS
Most often, infection is caused by *Proteus mirabilis*, but other bacteria may also be present so that the typical histology is not related to any specific organism.

CLINICAL HISTORY AND PHYSICAL EXAMINATION
Xanthogranulomatous pyelonephritis usually presents with loin pain, fever, weight loss, and general malaise. A renal mass may be palpable.

DIFFERENTIAL DIAGNOSIS
Renal cell carcinoma and renal tuberculosis are the main differential diagnoses.

INVESTIGATIONS
Urinalysis shows pyuria and microscopic hematuria. Urine culture is usually positive. Anemia, leucocytosis and abnormal liver function tests are often found. Intravenous urography shows an enlarged kidney usually associated wiith calculi; the kidney is usually nonfunctional, but calyceal distortion may be evident. CT demonstrates multiple low attenuation areas of soft tissue density within the kidney surrounded by thickened parenchyma (**143**). Biopsy and culture may be necessary to confirm the diagnosis.

HISTOLOGY
The kidney is enlarged. The cut surface appears yellow and there may be multiple abscesses. There is inflammation around the kidney. The yellow areas consist of sheets of large foamy lipid-containing macrophages, neutrophils, plasma cells, and necrotic debris (**144**).

PROGNOSIS AND MANAGEMENT
Usually irreversible renal damage has been done by the time of diagnosis and nephrectomy is the treatment of choice. Fortunately subsequent involvement of the contralateral kidney does not seem to occur.

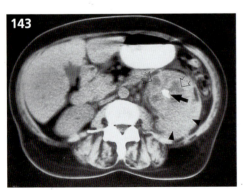

143 CT scan in a patient with xanthogranulomatous pyelonephritis affecting the left kidney. There is a calculus in the lower pole of the left kidney (arrow) with a soft tissue inflammatory mass surrounding the posterior aspect of the left lower pole (arrowheads). Also note the low-density lipid (open arrows) replacing the parenchyma of the left kidney.

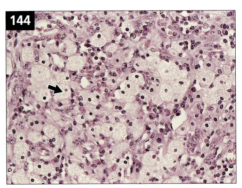

144 Xanthogranulomatous pyelonephritis. Large numbers of foamy lipid laden macrophages (arrow). Light microscopy (H+E x400).

Malakoplakia

DEFINITION
Malakoplakia is a rare condition which usually affects the bladder but can affect the ureters and kidneys. It is characterized by aggregates of macrophages containing inclusion bodies.

EPIDEMIOLOGY AND ETIOLOGY
It is more common in females and the elderly.

PATHOGENESIS
Malakoplakia is usually associated with *E.coli* infection, and is thought to be a result of a defect in bactericidal function of macrophages.

CLINICAL HISTORY AND PHYSICAL EXAMINATION
Lower urinary tract malakoplakia usually presents with urinary frequency, urgency or hematuria. Renal malakoplakia may present with renal impairment and fever.

DIFFERENTIAL DIAGNOSIS
This is similar to xanthogranulomatous pyelonephritis.

INVESTIGATIONS
Renal imaging will often show enlarged kidneys. Histology is necessary to make a diagnosis.

HISTOLOGY (145–147)
The renal parenchyma is replaced by collections of large macrophages. These may contain round, laminated, basophilic bodies termed Michaelis–Gutman bodies.

PROGNOSIS
Untreated renal impairment will progress, but after treatment with antibiotics renal function will stabilize or improve.

MANAGEMENT
Treatment is with a 6-week course of antibiotics followed by low-dose prophylaxis for at least 12 months. There is some evidence for Vitamin C and cholinergic agents being of benefit.

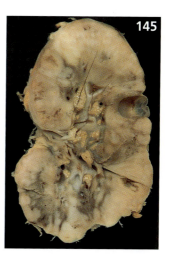

145 Gross specimen of malakoplakia. The cut surface contains cream-colored nodules surrounded by normal parenchyma. Microscopy of the nodules shows malakoplakia.

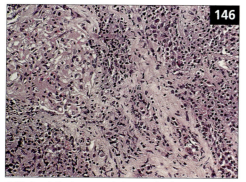

146 A relatively normal glomerulus is seen top right; tubules are replaced by a dense mononuclear cell infiltrate, rich in plasma cells. Light microscopy (H+E ×250).

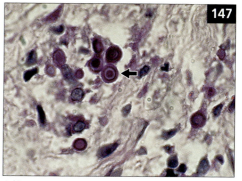

147 High power micrograph showing numerous Michaelis–Gutman bodies (arrow). Light microscopy (PAS ×1000).

Renal tuberculosis

DEFINITION
About 20% of all cases of extrapulmonary tuberculosis involve the genitourinary tract. In the West, most cases are due to *Mycobacterium tuberculosis*.

EPIDEMIOLOGY AND ETIOLOGY
Renal tuberculosis is more common in men, and has a peak incidence in the fifth decade. There is a latent period of months to decades between the primary infection and diagnosis of renal tuberculosis. Since the 1980s the incidence has been increasing, partly due to the AIDS epidemic. About 4–8% of patients with pulmonary tuberculosis will develop genitourinary tuberculosis.

PATHOGENESIS
Following the transmission of tuberculous infection by inhalation or ingestion, a primary focus develops which usually heals spontaneously. However, the primary infection often causes a silent bacillemia which seeds to the kidneys amongst other organs, leading to bilateral granulomatous glomerular involvement. As delayed hypersensitivity develops, these lesions may resolve or progress slowly by rupturing into the tubular lumen and causing medullary granulomas. These lesions caseate producing tumor-like masses called tuberculomas, cavitating lesions and calyceal amputation (**148**). Seeding of the urine may result in involvement of the urothelium of the renal pelvis, ureter, and bladder as well as the genital organs.

CLINICAL HISTORY AND PHYSICAL EXAMINATION
Considerable tissue destruction may have occurred before symptoms develop. Some patients are asymptomatic and are diagnosed during the investigation of sterile pyuria. In symptomatic patients, the commonest symptoms are frequency, dysuria, loin pain, and hematuria. Constitutional symptoms are usually slight. Physical examination is often unremarkable.

DIFFERENTIAL DIAGNOSIS
The differential diagnosis of the symptoms of lower urinary tract disease includes acute bacterial infections and neoplasia. The differential of a renal mass includes renal cell carcinoma and xanthogranulomatous pyelonephritis.

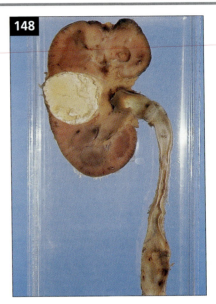

148

INVESTIGATIONS
Urinalysis shows sterile pyuria and microscopic hematuria. Renal impairment is rare unless there is bilateral ureteric stricturing. The key test is urine culture of early-morning urine samples. Abdominal X-ray may show renal calcification. Intravenous urography at an early stage of disease shows calyceal blunting, and at a later stage destruction of the papillae and multiple ureteric strictures. CT is useful in the investigation of a nonfunctioning kidney. Renal biopsy is not usually indicated, but histology will show a caseating interstitial nephritis (**149, 150**).

PROGNOSIS
Complications include formation of abscess cavities which may become secondarily infected with pyogenic organisms, hemorrhage, and fistula formation. Renal failure may result from bilateral obstruction. Hypertension may be caused by a nonfunctioning kidney.

MANAGEMENT
Genitourinary infections by sensitive organisms are treated with 6 months of isoniazid and rifampin (rifampicin), and pyrazinamide for the first 2 months. If the organism is isoniazid resistant, at least four drugs are given. Progressive ureteric strictures require reconstructive surgery. Nephrectomy may be indicated for sepsis, hemorrhage, intractable pain, inability to sterilize the urine with drugs, and new onset severe hypertension.

148 Opposite. Late caseous and ulcerative tuberculosis. Cut surface shows middle calyceal system completely replaced by a tuberculous abscess containing chalky caseous pus. The upper pole shows scarring and cavitation. The ureter is distended with a stricture at the lower end.

149 Tuberculosis showing widespread tubular destruction with a caseating granuloma and a Langerhans giant cell (arrow). Light microscopy (H+E ×150).

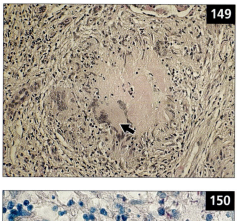

150 Ziehl-Neelsen stained section showing acid fast bacilli (arrows). Light microscopy (Ziehl-Neelson ×400).

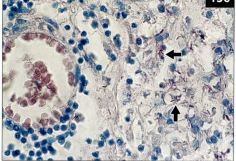

Two unusual renal infections

SYPHILITIC GUMMA OF KIDNEY (151)

HYDATID CYST OF KIDNEY (152)

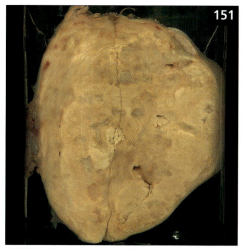

151 The kidney is occupied by a massive gumma in which irregular caseous zones of gummatous necrosis lie embedded in dense scar tissue. Microscopy shows necrosis with infiltrating lymphocytes and macrophages.

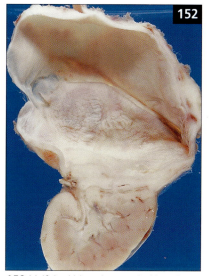

152 Half the kidney is occupied by a large, opened leathery cyst, the external capsule, from which the internal hydatid has been removed.

Vesicoureteric reflux and reflux nephropathy

DEFINITION

Primary vesicoureteric reflux is a common congenital condition with a probable autosomal dominant inheritance with variable penetrance. The end result is reflux nephropathy which may present with urinary tract infections, hypertension, proteinuria, or renal impairment.

Reflux nephropathy has replaced the term 'chronic nonobstructive atrophic pyelonephritis' to describe the small, irregularly-scarred kidney which occurs in this condition. This is a better name because it recognizes the importance of vesicoureteric reflux, and does not imply bacterial infection, the role of which is controversial.

EPIDEMIOLOGY AND ETIOLOGY

Studies of affected families suggest a single autosomal dominant gene to be reponsible for vesicoureteric reflux. The gene for this condition remains to be discovered. The prevalence of primary vesicoureteric reflux is uncertain. Studies vary from 0.4–9.0% of the otherwise normal infant population. Reflux nephropathy is probably responsible for about 10% of patients reaching end-stage renal failure. These patients usually require renal replacement therapy in the second or third decade.

PATHOGENESIS

Primary vesicoureteric reflux is the backflow of urine through the vesicoureteric junction (VUJ) due to shortness of the submucosal segment of ureter, probably as a result of congenital lateral ectopia of the ureteric orifice. As a child grows the intravesical ureter lengthens and reflux decreases with age. Renal damage is associated with intrarenal reflux; urine under high pressure is forced back up the collecting ducts. This may be sufficient to initiate the scarring process. Bacterial infection probably accelerates the scarring. Much of the damage caused by reflux occurs *in utero* or in the first months of life. Another theory is that the abnormal renal development is a form of renal dysplasia.

CLINICAL HISTORY AND PHYSICAL EXAMINATION

Reflux nephropathy may present with recurrent urinary tract infections, nocturnal enuresis, hypertension, proteinuria, renal impairment, or with asymmetric kidneys on renal imaging.

INVESTIGATIONS

Fetal ultrasonography can detect hydronephrosis *in utero* and neonates who have persistent upper tract dilatation should have micturating cystourethography performed. This can be performed with radiologic contrast (**153**) or radionuclides. These techniques allow assessment of the severity of reflux. Intravenous urography is the traditional method for imaging reflux nephropathy. There is usually reduced renal size, and localized thinning of the renal parenchyma associated with clubbing and dilatation of the directly underlying calyx due to contraction of the renal papilla (**154**). DMSA scans are very sensitive for detecting scars and also reliably measure single kidney function (**155**).

HISTOLOGY

The macroscopic features are of coarse segmental scarring (**156**), most prominent at the poles. The scars are related to the dilated calyx. In the scarred areas there is tubulointerstitial fibrosis and often a lymphocytic infiltrate. In other areas there may be appearances of focal and segmental glomerulosclerosis which is a result of glomerular hyperfiltration in the remnant nephrons.

PROGNOSIS

Some kidneys subjected to vesicoureteric reflux will become progressively damaged, whereas others will be unaffected. The severity of reflux is the major risk factor for renal parenchymal damage.

MANAGEMENT

Children with vesicoureteric reflux should be placed on long-term antibiotic prophylaxis as this has been shown to reduce progression to renal failure. In general surgery has not been shown to be of benefit except in the most severe grades of reflux. Siblings of affected children should be screened for the condition.

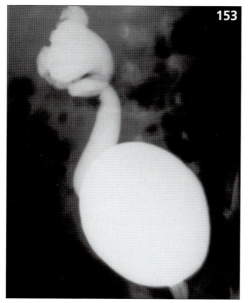

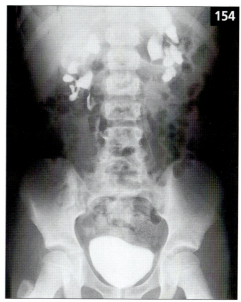

153 Micturating cystourethrogram showing gross unilateral reflux.

154 Intravenous pyelogram of a 9-year-old female presenting with recurrent urinary tract infections. Bilateral vesicoureteric reflux is present, with cortical scarring and calyceal dilatation.

155 DMSA scan showing bilateral severe renal scarring.

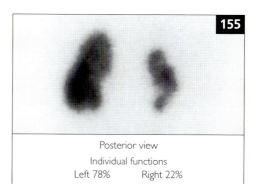

Posterior view

Individual functions

Left 78%   Right 22%

156 Chronic pyelonephritis. The kidneys are unequal in size, with scarring of the cortex.

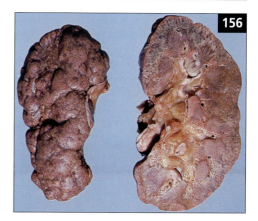

Urinary tract obstruction

DEFINITION
Obstructive uropathy describes the structural changes in the urinary tract that impair outflow of urine. Obstructive nephropathy refers to the renal disease that results from impaired flow of urine. Hydronephrosis refers to dilatation of the renal pelvis; it may occur in the absence of obstruction, for example in vesicoureteric reflux or pregnancy. Obstruction may be acute, for example due to a stone, or sloughed papilla or chronic, e.g. due to congenital conditions.

Obstruction as a cause of acute renal failure (ARF) is covered in Chapter 10, p. 170.

EPIDEMIOLOGY AND ETIOLOGY
Obstructive uropathy is most common at the extremes of life. In early childhood it is a result of congenital abnormalities of the urinary tract. In elderly men it is usually due to prostatic disease. Obstruction may be caused by lesions within the lumen or the wall of the urinary tract or by extrinsic compression (*Table 8*).

PATHOGENESIS
Acute obstruction leads to increased ureteric pressure, and briefly increased renal blood flow before this declines. The kidney becomes edematous and hemorrhagic. Histologically there is tubular dilatation. Chronic obstruction causes thinning of the renal parenchyma probably as a result of raised back-pressure and renal ischemia, and dilatation of the renal pelvis. Histologically there is tubulointerstitial fibrosis, dilated tubules, and global sclerosis of some glomeruli. If bacterial infection is present rapid destruction of the renal substance can occur.

CLINICAL HISTORY AND PHYSICAL EXAMINATION
Acute upper tract obstruction causes pain in the loin which typically radiates to the groin. Pain is exacerbated by a high fluid intake, alcohol, or diuretics. In children the kidney may be palpable. In the presence of infection there is fever and increased loin tenderness. Complete anuria develops only if there is complete bilateral obstruction of a single functioning kidney. If obstruction is incomplete there may be polyuria. In the presence of intermittent obstruction there may be alternating polyuria and anuria. Lower tract obstruction usually causes hesitancy in starting urination, weak stream, terminal dribbling, and acute urinary retention. Chronic obstruction may be asymptomatic and patients present with renal failure. Repeated urinary tract infections, especially in a male, should raise the possibility of obstruction. Hypertension is common in acute and chronic obstruction.

DIFFERENTIAL DIAGNOSIS
The differential of complete anuria includes severe acute glomerulonephritis and bilateral renal arterial occlusion.

INVESTIGATIONS
Ultrasound is the first-line investigation as it is noninvasive and will detect dilatation of the renal pelvis (**157**). It does not distinguish between dilated obstructed systems and nonobstructed distended systems. Furthermore, not all cases of acute obstruction will have dilated systems.

Plain abdominal X-rays with tomograms will detect radio-opaque stones (90%). Intravenous urography may help to define the site, degree, and cause of obstruction (**158**) but care needs to be taken in patients with renal impairment, myeloma, and diabetes mellitus because of the nephrotoxicity of radiocontrast dye. In cases of acute obstruction the obstructed kidney is enlarged and smooth in outline, the nephrogram is delayed and dense, and the ureter may be dilated down to the level of obstruction. In long-standing obstruction there is generalized thinning of the renal parenchyma and calyceal dilatation. Spiral CT is sensitive for detection of renal calculi and CT is necessary to define retroperitoneal and pelvic lesions.

Furosemide (frusemide) renography is helpful in distinguishing between a nonobstructed dilated collecting system and true obstruction (**159, 160**).

PROGNOSIS
This clearly depends on the site, duration and cause of obstruction. Infection will rapidly destroy the renal parenchyma.

MANAGEMENT
If infection is present, obstruction must be relieved immediately, usually by the insertion of a percutaneous antegrade nephrostomy, and broad-spectrum antibiotics. Stones of <5 mm (0.2 in) usually pass spontaneously. About 50% of 5–7 mm (0.2–0.3 in) stones will pass. Larger stones require intervention either by lithotripsy or endourological techniques. Patients with PUJ obstruction are treated by Anderson Hynes

pyeloplasty. In patients with malignant disease, decisions are made on an individual basis about the appropriateness of intervention.

Table 8 Causes of urinary obstruction

Within the lumen
Calculus
Sloughed papilla
Blood clot
Fungus balls

Within the wall
PUJ obstruction
VUJ obstruction
Strictures (TB, calculi)
Ureteric, bladder tumors
Neurogenic bladder
Posterior urethral valves
Ureterocele
Urethral stricture

Extrinsic compression
Retroperitoneal fibrosis
Retroperitoneal tumors
Iatrogenic (ligation)
Prostatic disease
Cervical carcinoma
Crohn's disease

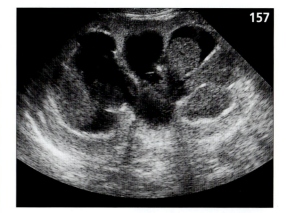

157 Ultrasound. Hydronephrosis is seen with echogenic fungal balls within the dilated calyces.

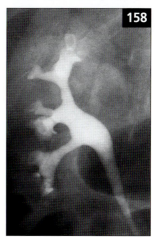

158 Papillary necrosis (from analgesic abuse). Intravenous urogram reveals small collections of contrast material of various sizes in the papillae of the right kidney.

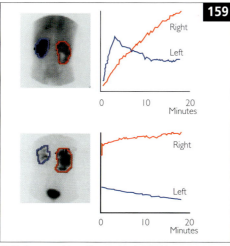

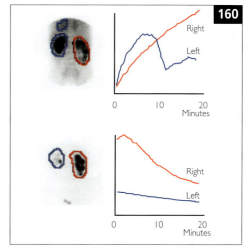

159 Furosemide- (frusemide-) DTPA renogram demonstrating right pelviureteric junction obstruction. The upper panel pre-frusemide, and the lower panel post-frusemide. There is no drainage from the right renal pelvis.

160 Furosemide- (frusemide-) DTPA renogram demonstrating a baggy but nonobstructed right renal pelvis. The upper panel pre-frusemide, and the lower panel post-frusemide.

Congenital anomalies of the urinary tract

Malformations of the urinary tract are among the most common of all congenital anomalies. They vary in severity from noncompatability with life, e.g. bilateral renal agenesis, to often asymptomatic anomalies, e.g. horseshoe kidney. Congenital abnormalities of the kidney and urinary tract are listed (*Table 9*), and certain types are illustrated in **161–168**.

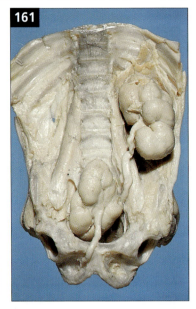

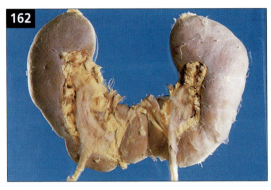

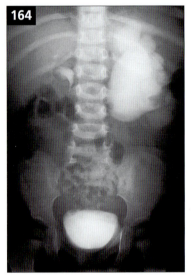

161 Pelvic ectopia. A portion of the trunk of a fetus dissected to show the right kidney lying upon the vertebral column at the pelvic brim. The ureter arises from the anterior aspect of the organ. The left kidney and adrenal gland are in normal position. Most pelvic kidneys are asymptomatic, but may develop pyelonephritis or be the cause of an obstructed delivery.

162 Horseshoe kidney, present in 1:500 autopsies. The total amount of renal substance is within normal limits, but there is continuity between the lower poles of each kidney anterior to the aorta. The pelvis looks directly forward and ureters pass superficial to the median communicating bridge of renal tissue.

163 Unilateral renal dysplasia in a 1-month-old child. Kidney is occupied by large numbers of translucent, variably sized cysts. Unilateral renal dysplasia is the commonest abnormal abdominal mass palpable in neonates. There is no mature renal tissue. It is comprised of undifferentiated mesenchyme from which abortive tubules and primitive glomeruli are formed. Some tubules show cystic dilatation. Nodules of cartilage and bone may be present.

164 Intravenous pyelogram showing left pelviureteric junction obstruction.

165 Duplex pelvis and kidney. Bisected adult kidney of normal size with separate pelvicalyceal systems at each pole, each draining via a separate ureter which fuse later in the course. The single ureter enters the bladder normally. Duplex pelvis/ureter is the commonest congenital abnormality of the renal collecting system with some degree of duplication found in 4–6% autopsies. It varies from mere extrarenal bifurcation of the pelvis, to replication of the entire course of the ureter with two openings into the bladder.

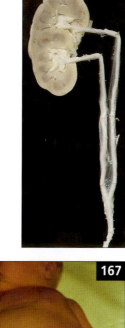

166 Posterior urethral valves. Both kidneys are massively enlarged and hydronephrotic. The bladder and ureters are distended with almost complete obstruction of the membranous urethra.

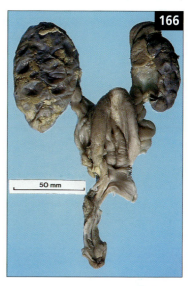

167 Prune belly syndrome: baby showing lack of abdominal musculature.

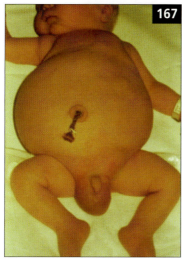

168 Micturating cystourethrogram in the same child as **167** showing megaureters and megacystis.

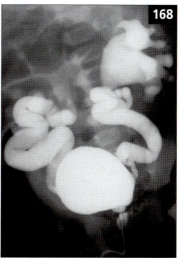

Table 9 Congenital abnormalities of the kidney and urinary tract

Renal abnormalities
Agenesis (unilateral or bilateral)
Hypoplasia (oligomeganephronia,
    segmental [Ask–Upmark kidney])
Ectopia (simple, crossed, horseshoe)
Dysplasia

Ureteric abnormalities
Atresia
Duplication
Ectopic
Ureterocoele
Vesicoureteric reflux

Bladder abnormalities
Urachus
Exstrophy

Urethral abnormalities
Valves
Hypospadias

Renal calculi

Renal calculi may occur in 12% of the population. They are more common in males, and the highest incidence is seen in the fifth and sixth decades. Sixty to seventy per cent of stones consist of calcium oxalate alone or calcium oxalate together with calcium phosphate. Pure calcium phosphate stones occur in about 7%. About 10–20% of stones are made of magnesium ammonium phosphate hexahydrate (struvite) together with carbonate apatite and are a result of urinary infection by bacteria producing urease which alkalinize the urine. Uric acid stones make up 5–10% of all stones and cystine stones 1–2%.

Stones may be asymptomatic and discovered by chance when renal imaging is performed. Renal colic occurs when the stone passes down the ureter. The pain resolves immediately the stone passes. Loin pain and fever occur when there is obstruction and infection.

CALCIUM STONE DISEASE
Definition
Calcium-containing stones are the commonest renal calculi.

Epidemiology and etiology
The main risk factors in calcium stone disease are a low urinary volume and low pH, a high excretion of calcium, oxalate, and uric acid, and a low level of inhibitors of crystal formation. Underlying diseases which predispose to stone formation include primary hyperparathyroidism, enteric hyperoxaluria, primary hyperoxaluria, renal tubular acidosis, Cushing's syndrome, vitamin D intoxication, immobilization, milk-alkali syndrome, and medullary sponge kidney. The majority of stones are idiopathic. Hyperoxaluria seems to be a more important risk factor than hypercalciuria. Recurrent stones are common.

Pathogenesis
The initial stage is crystal formation due to supersaturation of the urine. Calcium phosphate may form a nucleus for calcium oxalate crystallization. Stones may become anchored at the calyceal tip of renal papillae allowing the stones to grow.

Clinical history
Calcium stones may be asymptomatic and discovered only on coincidental imaging, or may present with the passage of a single stone or gravel every few days, or with ureteral obstruction.

Investigations
Radiodense stones are seen on X-ray and spiral CT (**169**). Calcium oxalate/phosphate crystals may be seen in the sediment from fresh warm urine (**170**). A 24-hour urinary collection should be performed and volume, calcium, creatinine, urate, and oxalate measured.

Management
Patients are advised to drink enough fluid to allow a urine flow of >3 l of urine per day. Foods rich in oxalate should be avoided (rhubarb, nuts, strawberries, raspberries, tea, and chocolate). Thiazides lower urinary calcium excretion.

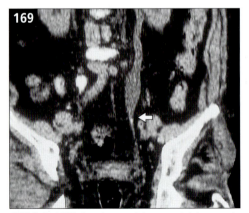

169 Spiral CT showing a calcium-containing renal calculus (arrow).

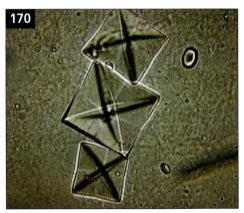

170 Urine microscopy showing calcium oxalate crystals (×400).

INFECTION STONES

Definition
The typical infection stone contains magnesium ammonium phosphate (struvite) and calcium phosphate in roughly equal amounts, together with carbonate.

Epidemiology and etiology
The most usual organisms are *Proteus mirabilis*, *Escherischia coli*, or *Klebsiella*. These bacteria split urea to ammonia and carbon dioxide which leads to alkaline urine leading to precipitation of calcium phosphate and magnesium ammonium phosphate. These stones are more common in females and patients with structurally abnormal urinary tracts in whom urinary infections are more common. Very large stones may be formed and have the shape of the renal pelvis and calyces (staghorn calculi) (**171**). These stones harbor infection and lead to pyelonephritis and renal damage.

Clinical history
Most patients have recurrent urinary tract infections. The stones may be asymptomatic or cause recurrent loin pain and fever.

Investigations
The urine is alkaline and there is minor proteinuria. White cells, bacilli, and struvite crystals are found on urine microscopy. Urine culture is usually positive. Plain radiographs demonstrate the stones.

Management
Treatment is with surgery or shock-wave lithotripsy to eliminate the stones and correct any anatomic abnormality. Appropriate antibiotic coverage must be given. When stone fragments remain, infection persists and new stones are frequent.

URIC ACID STONES

Definition
Uric acid stones are formed as a result of either uric acid overproduction and hyperuricosuria (>4.5 mmol [75.6 mg.dl]/day), a low urine volume (<1 l) or a persistently acidic urine (<pH 5.5).

Epidemiology and etiology
Uric acid stones occur most frequently in middle-aged males. Most cases are idiopathic associated with low urinary pH. Uric acid stones are most common in Western populations who have a high purine intake. Uric acid stones may occur in patients with gout and patients who develop hyperuricemia following chemotherapy. Patients with diarrheal diseases or an ileostomy have a metabolic acidosis which predisposes to stone formation.

Clinical history
Symptoms vary from the occasional passage of gravel to acute ureteral obstruction.

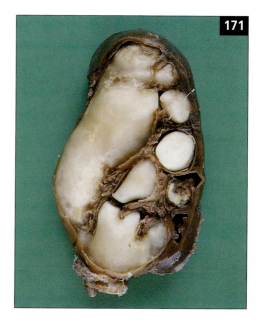

171 Anterior half of kidney has been removed to display a large staghorn calculus which has destroyed most of the kidney.

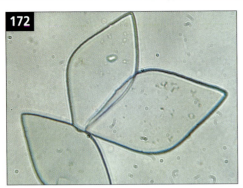

172 Urine microscopy containing uric acid crystals (×200).

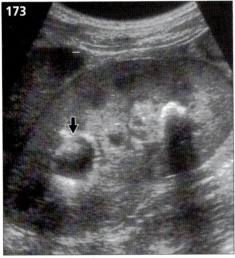

173 Echogenic shadows caused by uric acid stones (arrow).

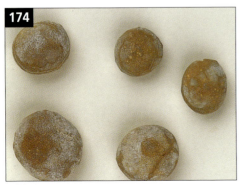

174 Urate stones.

Renal calculi (*continued*)

Investigations
Urine pH is usually <5.5, and uric acid crystals are seen in a fresh urine sample (**172**). The stones are radiolucent on intravenous urography, but are detected by ultrasound (**173, 174**).

Management
High water intake together with alkali and allopurinol is effective not only in preventing new stone formation but also in dissolving stones.

CYSTINURIA
Definition
Cystinuria is a hereditary disorder of cystine and dibasic amino acid (lysine, ornithine, arginine) transport resulting in formation of cystine stones.

Epidemiology and etiology
The disease is inherited as autosomal recessive. The incidence varies from 1:15,000 in the US to 1:2500 in Libyan Jews. It affects both genders with equal frequency, but is more severe in males. Cystine urolithiasis accounts for 1% to 2% of patients with renal calculi in the US. Two cystinuria genes have been identified. The rBAT gene has been mapped to chromosome 2p21. rBAT expression is present in the straight (S3) portion of the renal proximal tubule and small intestine. Over 30 distinct rBAT mutations have been described and account for patients with type I cystinuria (fully recessive). The second cystinuria gene (SLC7A9) has been localized on chromosome 19q. Mutations in SLC7A9 account for the incompletely recessive forms of cystinuria (types II and III).

Pathogenesis
In humans, 99% of cystine in the glomerular filtrate is normally reabsorbed by transporters located in the luminal brush border membrane of cells of the proximal tubule. In patients with cystinuria, a defect of the transepithelial transport of cystine and dibasic amino acids in the proximal renal tubule results in urinary excretion of cystine which usually exceeds 400 mg/24 h (>50–200% the normal filtered load). Cystine is the least soluble of all amino acids. At a urinary pH between 5.0 and 7.0, cystine precipitates in the urine when concentration levels increase above 300 mg/l. Current evidence suggests that the SLC7A9 gene encodes for a transmembrane channel protein that mediates cystine and dibasic amino acids uptake at the luminal surface. The smaller rBAT protein forms a heterodimeric complex

with this channel and appears critical for its targeting to the luminal membrane.

Clinical history

The disease is usually first manifested by the development of symptomatic urolithiasis in a teenager or young adult. However, there have been reports of infants and octogenarians presenting with cystine calculi. Patients commonly have multiple cystine calculi or large staghorn calculi. Urinary tract obstruction and infection are a common association and the causes of chronic renal failure in these patients.

Differential diagnosis

The differential diagnosis is with other causes of stone formation. Cystinuria has also been described to occur as part of a syndrome associated with hyperuricemia and uric acid stones. The diagnosis of urolithiasis in a child or history of recurrent urolithiasis should prompt the evaluation for cystinuria.

Investigations

Examination of acid urine shows the typical cystine crystals, which appear as hexagonal, flat structures (175). Pure cystine stones appear yellow-brown to sand-colored and granular. Because of their high sulfur content, pure cystine stones are radiopaque (176). Frequently, however, cystine stones undergo calcium oxalate, calcium phosphate, and magnesium ammonium phosphate deposition. Urine electrophoresis or chromatography can be used to identify lysine, arginine, and ornithine in increased quantities in the urine.

Management

The goal of therapy is to reduce the concentration of cystine in the urine below supersaturation levels to prevent precipitation, and stone formation. The solubility of cystine is constant within the range of urinary pH 5.0–7.0 (250 mg/l), but increases significantly at urinary pH above 7.5 (500 mg/l). Thus, increasing fluid intake and alkalinization of the urine are the major therapeutic maneuvers. Fluid intake large enough to maintain a daily urine volume of >3 l requires overnight hydration, but is essential for therapeutic success. For alkalinizing the urine, potassium citrate supplements, rather than sodium bicarbonate, should be used since sodium restriction lowers urinary cystine content. Administration of thiol derivates such as D-penicillamine and α-mercaptopropionylglycine, cleave cystine into 2 cysteine moieties and combine with a molecule of cysteine to form a highly-soluble disulfide compound decreasing the excretion of cystine. Because of their toxicity profile, these agents should be reserved for patients in whom increased fluid intake and urinary alkalinization are insufficient to prevent formation of new or dissolution of pre-existing stones. Frequent clinical, radiological, and laboratory surveillance are important to identify complications (e.g. obstruction), and to keep patients motivated and maintain long-term compliance with therapy. Cystine stones are poorly fragmented by extracorporeal shock-wave lithotripsy. Relief of urinary tract obstruction frequently requires surgical manipulation.

Prognosis

The prognosis is usually good for patients compliant with a high fluid intake and urine alkalinization. However, recurrent urinary tract obstruction and infection will result in some patients developing end-stage renal failure. For these patients, renal transplantation is the treatment of choice.

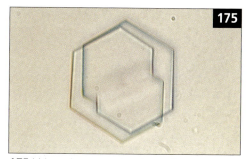

175 Urine microscopy showing cystine stones (×200).

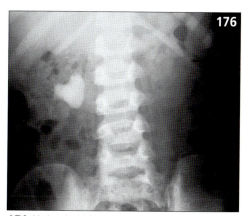

176 Abdominal X-ray showing a large cystine stone.

Retroperitoneal fibrosis

DEFINITION
Idiopathic retroperitoneal fibrosis (RPF) is a rare condition in which the ureters in their middle thirds become embedded in dense fibrous tissue, pulled towards the midline and extrinsic obstruction occurs.

EPIDEMIOLOGY AND ETIOLOGY
The condition is three times more common in males than in females. Peak incidence is in the fifth decade. Some cases may be related to inflammatory abdominal aortic aneurysms. There is a rare association with mediastinal fibrosis. Certain drugs such as methysergide, beta-blockers, and methyldopa have been implicated.

PATHOGENESIS
The periaortic fibrosis may represent an autoimmune response to leakage of material from atheromatous plaques in the diseased aorta.

CLINICAL HISTORY AND EXAMINATION
Patients may complain of loin or back pain (**269, 270**). The patient is often hypertensive with significant renal impairment. A hydrocele is found in 10% of patients.

DIFFERENTIAL DIAGNOSIS
The differential of a retroperitoneal mass causing ureteric obstruction includes lymphoma and carcinoma. A biopsy of the mass is necessary to make a definitive diagnosis.

INVESTIGATIONS
The ESR is usually raised and there is often a normochromic normocytic anemia. CT will define the peri-aortic mass (**177**). Biopsy is usually done at the time of ureterolysis, or under CT guidance.

PROGNOSIS
Renal prognosis is worse in cases of bilateral obstruction, which present with advanced renal failure.

MANAGEMENT
Surgical treatment is by ureterolysis. Corticosteroids will cause the peri-aortic mass to shrink. Relapse is possible after stopping steroid therapy. Life-long follow-up is necessary.

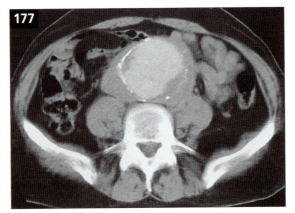

177 Retroperitoneal fibrosis. CT showing an inflammatory aortic aneurysm causing bilateral ureteric obstruction.

Medullary sponge kidney

DEFINITION

Medullary sponge kidney is due to dilatation of the inner medullary collecting ducts with enlargement of the pyramids, giving a spongy appearance to the kidney (**178**).

EPIDEMIOLOGY AND ETIOLOGY

A few cases are familial but most cases are sporadic. There is a definite association with congenital hemihypertrophy. The pathogenesis is unknown. It affects both sexes and presents usually between 20–45 years.

CLINICAL HISTORY

Medullary sponge kidney usually presents as a result of urinary tract infection or calcium stone formation. Renal colic and macroscopic hematuria are common. Renal function is normal although there may be decreased urinary concentrating ability and distal renal tubular acidosis.

DIFFERENTIAL DIAGNOSIS

This includes nephrocalcinosis, renal tuberculosis, papillary necrosis, and medullary cystic disease.

INVESTIGATIONS

Intravenous urography is the diagnostic procedure. In florid cases there is cystic dilatation of the collecting ducts, giving the 'bunch of grapes' appearance. There may be stones in the enlarged papillae (**179**). Ultrasound will show renal calcification.

PROGNOSIS

Progression to end-stage renal failure is rare. However, some patients may suffer considerable morbidity from the continuous passage of stones and may become dependent on analgesics.

MANAGEMENT

A high fluid intake and thiazides for patients with hypercalciuria are recommended.

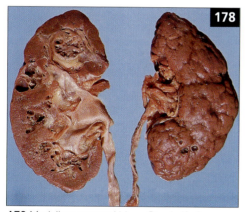

178 Medullary sponge kidney. One-half of each kidney is shown. Marked scarring of the subcapsular surface is present. Multiple minute cysts in the medullary pyramids give the cut surface the appearance of a sponge.

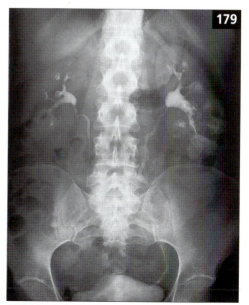

179 Intravenous pyelogram of a medullary sponge kidney.

Chapter Seven

Inherited renal diseases

- **Autosomal dominant polycystic kidney disease**

- **Autosomal recessive polycystic kidney disease**

- **Nephronophthisis (autosomal recessive juvenile nephronophthisis)**

- **Alport's syndrome**

- **Nail–patella syndrome**

- **Congenital nephrotic syndrome**

- **Fabry disease (Anderson–Fabry disease, angiokeratoma corporis diffusum)**

- **Von Hippel–Lindau disease**

- **Primary hyperoxalurias (PH)**

- **Cystinosis**

- **Tuberous sclerosis complex (TSC)**

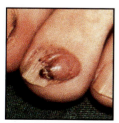
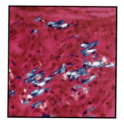
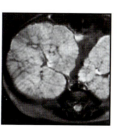
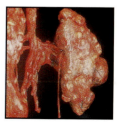

Autosomal dominant polycystic kidney disease

DEFINITION

Autosomal dominant polycystic kidney disease (ADPKD) is a genetically inherited systemic disorder characterized by multiple, bilateral renal cysts (**180**) associated with cysts in other organs such as liver and pancreas.

EPIDEMIOLOGY AND ETIOLOGY

ADPKD is a common disease with an incidence of 1:1,000 to 1:400. In the US alone there are approximately 400,000 patients with ADPKD and it is estimated that the disease is present in over 10 million patients worldwide. Both genders are affected. Mutations in at least two genes give rise to the disease. The PKD1 gene is on the short arm of chromosome 16 and is responsible for 85–90% of cases of ADPKD. The PKD2 gene maps to the long arm of chromosome 4. A third gene for ADPKD exists but its location is still unknown.

PATHOGENESIS

The PKD1 and PKD2 genes encode for two distinct proteins named polycystin 1 and polycystin 2, respectively. The PKD1 gene is a very large gene with 46 exons coding for 4302 amino acids. Computer modeling of polycystin 1 predicts a large extracellular N-terminal domain, multiple transmembrane loops, and a C-terminal intracellular tail (**181**). This structure suggests that polycystin 1 may function as a cell membrane receptor involved in cell–cell or cell–matrix interactions. The PKD2 gene contains 15 exons that code for 968 amino acids. Polycystin 2 contains an N-terminal cytoplasmic domain, six transmembrane domains, and a C-terminal cytoplasmic tail. The resulting protein has similarities to a voltage-activated calcium channel. It has been experimentally demonstrated that a tail-to-tail interaction may occur between polycystin 1 and polycystin 2, suggesting that the two proteins may function through a common signaling pathway. Although ADPKD is caused by an inherited germline mutation, only ~1% of nephrons will develop cysts. A two-hit hypothesis, in which a somatic mutation is superimposed on a germline mutation, has been postulated as the mechanism of cystogenesis in ADPKD.

The mechanism by which ADPKD causes renal failure is not clearly understood. It is likely to involve several mechanisms including compression of normal parenchyma by the cysts, hypertension, and production of inflammatory factors and growth factors by the cysts (angiotensin II, epidermal growth factor, osteopontin, transforming growth factor-β), resulting in interstitial inflammation and fibrosis.

CLINICAL HISTORY

The disease is characterized by multiple renal and extrarenal manifestations, but there is significant variability in the clinical presentation. Renal size increases with age with renal enlargement occurring in virtually all patients (**182–184**). Manifestations of renal involvement include pain, hematuria, hypertension, and renal insufficiency. Acute flank pain may occur as a result of cyst hemorrhage, infection, or stone. Macroscopic hematuria occurs in over 40% of patients with ADPKD and may be the presenting symptom. Cyst hemorrhage is frequent. It can present as macroscopic hematuria, or with pain and fever simulating infection of the cyst. In the majority of patients, symptoms resolve within 1 week. Persistence of hematuria, especially if the initial episode occurs after age 50 years, should prompt exclusion of underlying neoplasm. Urinary tract infection may present as cystitis, pyelonephritis, cyst infection, or a perinephric abscess. If cyst infection is suspected, cyst aspiration under ultrasound or CT guidance may need to be undertaken to confirm the diagnosis and guide selection of appropriate antimicrobial therapy.

Renal stones occur in approximately 20% of patients with ADPKD. In the majority of cases, the stones are composed of uric acid and/or calcium oxalate. CT scan is the procedure of choice to detect radiolucent stones and for differentiating stones from tumor or clots. An important complication of ADPKD is the development of hypertension. Hypertension precedes the development of renal failure. The prevalence of hypertension increases with age, affecting virtually all patients by the time renal failure develops. Patients with ADPKD are at an increased risk for early development of left ventricular hypertrophy and, therefore, are at increased risk for cardiovascular complications.

The most common extrarenal manifestation of ADPKD is polycystic liver disease (**185**). Multiple cysts result in hepatomegaly. Despite this, liver function is preserved. Females are more affected than males, particularly women who have had multiple pregnancies, suggesting that hepatic cyst growth is affected by estrogen. Massive liver enlargement can cause symptoms by compressing surrounding structures and include hepatic venous flow obstruction, inferior

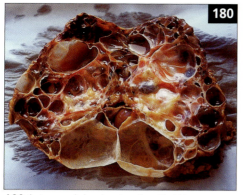

180 Autosomal dominant polycystic kidney disease. Gross specimen of a polycystic kidney.

181 Structural features of polycystin 1 and polycystin 2 molecules, and possible interaction of the molecules.

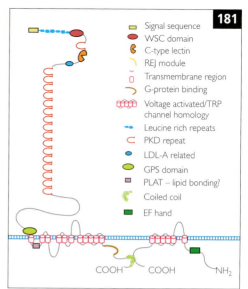

▭	Signal sequence
⬭	WSC domain
⟨	C-type lectin
⌒	REJ module
▯	Transmembrane region
⟩	G-protein binding
▥	Voltage activated/TRP channel homology
⇢	Leucine rich repeats
⊂	PKD repeat
●	LDL-A related
⬭	GPS domain
▪	PLAT – lipid bonding?
❦	Coiled coil
▬	EF hand

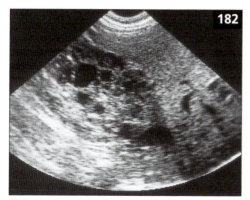

182 Autosomal dominant polycystic kidney disease. Ultrasound showing multiple cysts of different sizes.

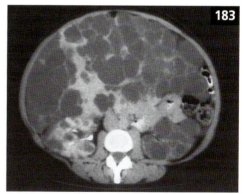

183 Autosomal dominant polycystic kidney disease. CT showing asymmetrically enlarged kidneys and polycystic liver.

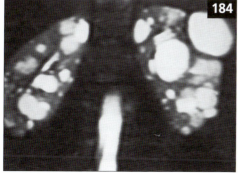

184 Autosomal dominant polycystic kidney disease. Renal MRI.

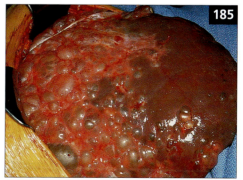

185 Large polycystic liver.

Autosomal dominant polycystic kidney disease (*continued*)

vena cava compression, and portal vein or bile duct compression. Treatment options to relieve the obstruction include aspiration of the cyst and alcohol sclerosis, laparoscopic fenestration, or combined hepatic resection and cyst fenestration. Other complications include cyst hemorrhage, infection, and rarely cyst rupture.

Another important extrarenal manifestation of ADPKD is the development of intracranial aneurysms. The incidence of the aneurysms varies according to the family history, occurring in approximately 5% of patients with a negative family history and 22% of those with a positive family history. The risk of rupture depends on the size of the aneurysm, being minimal for aneurysms <5 mm (0.2 in) in diameter but high for aneurysms >10 mm (0.4 in) in diameter. In addition to intracranial aneurysms, patients with ADPKD can present with other vascular abnormalities such as aneurysms of the thoracic aorta and coronary artery aneurysms. Other associated conditions include valvular heart abnormalities, most commonly mitral valve prolapse, pancreatic cysts, arachnoid cysts, spinal meningeal diverticula, and hernias.

PHYSICAL EXAMINATION
Hypertension is common. Renal size increases with age and kidneys become palpable in most cases. Liver enlargement, especially in women, may be found. Mitral or aortic regurgitation murmurs are commonly heard. Inguinal and umbilical hernias may be demonstrated.

DIFFERENTIAL DIAGNOSIS
The diagnosis is relatively straightforward in patients with a family history of ADPKD. In these patients, sonographic diagnostic criteria include two cysts arising unilaterally or bilaterally for individuals <30 years of age, two cysts in each kidney for individuals aged 30–59 years, and at least four cysts in each kidney for those over the age of 60 years. Presymptomatic screening by ultrasound before age 20 years is not recommended because results may not be conclusive. In patients without a family history the diagnosis is more difficult because of the variable clinical phenotype associated with ADPKD and because renal cystic disease can occur in other systemic diseases such as tuberous sclerosis complex, von Hippel–Lindau, and orofaciodigital syndrome type 1. Simple renal cysts are common, especially after the age of 50 years. Typically, these cysts are unilocular, and located in the renal cortex. Simple cysts are

often asymptomatic and are found incidentally on radiologic studies. Simple renal cysts must be distinguished from renal cell carcinoma. Multiple bilateral renal cysts are uncommon, and suggest an underlying inherited disease.

INVESTIGATIONS
In patients with a family history of ADPKD the diagnosis can be established using the renal ultrasonography criteria described above. Linkage genetic analysis can establish the diagnosis at the molecular level but requires other family members to be available for testing. It can also be used for prenatal diagnosis. Direct mutation analysis is possible in most families with PKD2. In patients with PKD1, direct mutation analysis is difficult because of the larger size of the gene and due to the fact that approximately 75% of the PKD1 gene is duplicated at least three times on chromosome 16.

HISTOLOGY
On gross examination, kidneys are enlarged and diffusely cystic. Microscopically, there is marked sclerosis of preglomerular vessels, interstitial fibrosis, and tubular epithelial hyperplasia (**186**). Interstitial fibrosis is an early finding, and is present even in patients with normal renal function. Microdissection studies demonstrate cysts arising from focal dilatation of renal tubules anywhere along the nephron. Epithelial cells lining the cysts are characterized by an increased nuclear to cytoplasmic ratio, decreased microvilli on the apical surface, reduced basolateral folding, and persistent expression of proteins present in earlier stages of development such as vimentin, clusterin, and PAX2. Microscopic adenomas have also been described.

PROGNOSIS
There is significant variability in the rate of progression of the renal disease, even within members of the same family. In approximately 50% of patients, end-stage renal failure occurs by the age of 55–75 years. Genetic and environmental factors appear to modulate the rate of progression of renal failure. The disease is usually milder in patients with mutations in the PKD2 gene than in patients with mutations in the PKD1 gene, who have an earlier onset of hypertension and progression to renal failure. Risk factors associated with progressive renal failure include PKD1 genotype, male gender, African-American background, early age at diagnosis (<30 years), and onset of hypertension

before age 35 years. Actuarial data indicate that ADPKD patients have a better dialysis outcome when compared with patients with end-stage renal failure from other causes.

MANAGEMENT

There is no specific treatment for patients with ADPKD. Current therapy is directed to controlling the renal and extrarenal complications of the disease. Uncontrolled hypertension accelerates the decline in renal function. Hypertension also aggravates target-organ damage, particularly left ventricular hypertrophy, and therefore should be tightly controlled. In some patients, large renal or liver cysts may require decompression, in order to control pain or complications from local compression (187, 188). Decompression of renal cysts does not affect the rate of progression to end-stage renal failure. Urinary tract infections or asymptomatic bacteriuria should be treated to prevent retrograde infection of the kidney. Infected cysts may require percutaneous or surgical drainage.

Screening for intracranial aneurysms is indicated in patients with a family history of aneurysm rupture, patients with a previous rupture, patients with high-risk occupations (e.g. pilots), development of symptoms, and patients who need reassurance. Magnetic resonance angiography is the screening method of choice. Surgical intervention is indicated for aneurysms ≥10 mm (0.4 in) in diameter. Hypertension, hyperlipidemia, and smoking are risk factors for rupture of intracranial aneurysm. Transplantation is the treatment of choice for patients who develop end-stage renal disease.

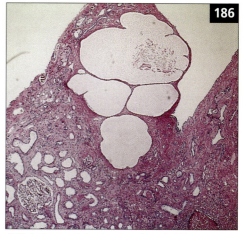

186 Autosomal dominant polycystic kidney disease. Light microscopy showing marked cystic dilatation of the tubules with severe interstitial fibrosis and tubular atrophy (H+E ×100).

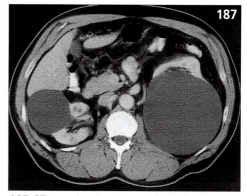

187 CT scan showing a large left renal cyst.

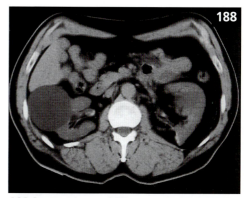

188 Same patient as **187**, post-cyst aspiration and ethanol ablation.

Autosomal recessive polycystic kidney disease

DEFINITION

Autosomal recessive polycystic kidney disease (ARPKD) is an inherited disease characterized by the association of polycystic kidneys with a biliary dysgenesis known as 'congenital hepatic fibrosis'.

EPIDEMIOLOGY AND ETIOLOGY

ARPKD has an estimated incidence of 1:20,000 live births. The genetic mutation has been mapped to the short arm of chromosome 6 (6p21-22). The polycystic kidney and hepatic disease 1 gene is a complex gene containing 67 exons, with several mRNAs generated by alternative splicing. The protein product (fibrocystin) is massive, containing 4074 amino acids (**189**). It contains a large highly glycosylated extracellular region, a single transmembrane domain and a short cytoplasmic tail containing potential phosphorylation sites. It is expressed in the collecting ducts of kidneys, bile ducts, and pancreas.

PATHOGENESIS

The biliary lesion is considered to be the result of an arrest in the normal organogenesis of the intrahepatic bile ducts, an abnormality termed ductal plate malformation. As a result, bile ducts persist in an embryonic form, the portal vein branches abnormally, and progressive portal fibrosis evolves. A similar maturational arrest mechanism has been postulated to occur in the kidney.

CLINICAL HISTORY

ARPKD affects both the kidneys and the liver. However, clinical presentation is extremely variable, even among members of the same family. The majority of patients present with large kidneys at birth or soon after (**190**). While cysts are present in 60–90% of their nephrons, liver involvement is mild. In other patients, the diagnosis is not made until after the third to the sixth month of life and can be as late as 1–5 years of age. In these patients, renal cysts involve only 10–25% of their nephrons, but hepatic fibrosis is severe. Occasionally, ARPKD can be diagnosed for the first time in a young adult. In neonates and young children, clinical manifestations that suggest the diagnosis include palpable abdominal masses, hypertension, and urinary tract infections. In older children, signs of hepatic involvement and portal hypertension predominate. Hypertension develops in over two-thirds of the patients. It usually begins within the first year of life, and can be severe. Abnormalities in urinary concentration are usually present but rarely cause clinical problems. The majority of patients have a slowly progressive

decrease in glomerular filtration rate, which starts at the same time as hypertension.

With progression of renal disease, kidneys tend to regress in size, and older patients may present with relatively small kidneys. Occasionally, large abdominal mass, oligohydramnios, and pulmonary hypoplasia (Potter syndrome) may be present at birth. Respiratory failure is the immediate cause of death in these patients. Liver involvement is a constant finding in patients with ARPKD. In contrast to the kidneys, liver cysts are not an important or common feature of ARPKD. Instead, hepatic involvement is secondary to fibrosis of the portal tracts and biliary dysgenesis. Hepatic involvement is clinically manifested by the signs of portal hypertension, usually occurring between 5 and 10 years of age. Hepatosplenomegaly, as well as hypersplenism, is usually found in these patients. In some cases, gross cystic dilatations of the intrahepatic biliary tree can simulate Caroli's disease. These patients are at increased risk of recurrent cholangitis.

PHYSICAL EXAMINATION

In neonates and young infants, palpable abdominal masses and hypertension are the signs that most often lead to the diagnosis. In older children and adolescents, hepatosplenomegaly and signs of portal hypertension predominate.

DIFFERENTIAL DIAGNOSIS

Although unusual, autosomal dominant polycystic kidney disease (ADPKD) can occur in infants and children, posing a diagnostic problem, especially in neonates. Family history, coupled with renal ultrasound of the parents, can help to establish the correct diagnosis. Other cystic diseases in children include renal cystic dysplasia, renal cysts associated with multiple malformation syndromes such as Meckel syndrome, Zellweger syndrome, Laurence–Moon–Biedl syndrome, several chromosomal disorders (trisomy 9, 13, 18, and 21), and the contiguous PKD1/TSC2 syndrome.

INVESTIGATIONS

Ultrasonography is the method of choice for initial screening. In neonates, renal ultrasound shows enlarged, hyperechogenic kidneys, with multiple small cysts in the cortex and in the medulla. In older children, larger cysts alter the renal contour and may simulate ADPKD. Ultrasound of the liver shows dilatation of the biliary ducts and signs of portal hypertension, but no cysts. Ultrasonography has also been used for antenatal screening. In severe cases, the use of this technique can lead to the diagnosis as early as week 16 of gestation.

However, mild forms may be missed. In families with other affected members, genetic linkage analysis can be used for prenatal diagnosis.

HISTOLOGY

The macroscopic appearance will depend on age at diagnosis. When ARPKD is diagnosed in the neonatal period, kidneys can have as much as ten times their expected weight. Despite their size, normal kidney shape is symmetrically maintained. Multiple 1–2 mm (0.04–0.08 in) cysts are visible at the tip of large cylindric or fusiform tubule channels that radiate from the calyxes through the entire cortical thickness. Dilated tubules are also seen in the medulla. In older patients (>1 year of age) the appearance of the kidneys changes. Fewer but larger cysts are present, giving the kidneys an overall bumpy and irregular appearance that may be indistinguishable from the pattern in ADPKD. Microscopically, neonatal kidneys are composed almost entirely of cystic tubules (**191**). There is strong evidence that the cysts originate from collecting ducts. Later on, the extent of cystic involvement decreases, but progressive glomerular sclerosis, tubular atrophy, and interstitial fibrosis develops.

PROGNOSIS

Neonates with severe disease usually die soon after birth from pulmonary insufficiency. Patients who survive the neonatal period usually have initially relatively well-preserved renal function. After the first few months, the course is variable. Some children will continue to have adequate renal function, while others will progress to end-stage renal failure. In general, progression of renal failure is slow and fewer than one-third of cases reach end-stage renal failure before adulthood. For children who survive the first year of life, recent series show a 60–80% probability of renal survival at 15 years. The prognosis for the liver involvement is related to the complications of portal hypertension since hepatocellular function remains normal long term. Effective management of portal hypertension, coupled with the widespread use of renal and liver transplantation, has resulted in significant improvement in long-term survival.

MANAGEMENT

Therapy is supportive and includes careful control of blood pressure. Renal transplantation is indicated for patients who develop end-stage renal disease. Portal hypertension needs close monitoring by serial ultrasound and Doppler flow studies. Esophageal varices may require banding or sclerotherapy. In some patients, portocaval or splenorenal shunt surgery is indicated. Patients with end-stage renal disease and severe portal hypertension are candidates for combined kidney and liver transplantation.

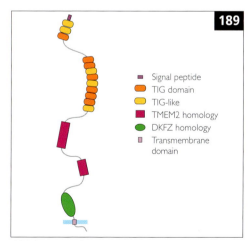

189 Structural features of fibrocystin, the autosomal recessive polycystic kidney disease molecule.

- Signal peptide
- TIG domain
- TIG-like
- TMEM2 homology
- DKFZ homology
- Transmembrane domain

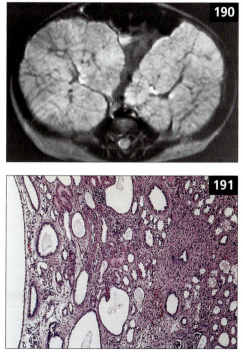

190 ARPKD. T2-weighted MRI of a 1-year old child showing massively enlarged kidneys.

191 ARPKD. Light microscopy showing cystic dilatation of the tubules (H+E ×100).

Nephronophthisis (autosomal recessive juvenile nephronophthisis)

DEFINITION
Juvenile nephronophthisis (NPH), also called nephronophthisis type 1 (NPH1), is an autosomal recessive disorder characterized by chronic tubulointerstitial nephritis and cysts at the corticomedullary border of the kidneys.

EPIDEMIOLOGY AND ETIOLOGY
At least three different loci for the disease have been identified, NPH1, NPH2, and NPH3, which correspond to three different forms of clinical presentation: juvenile, infantile, and adolescent respectively. NPH1 accounts for approximately 85% of cases of NPH, and is considered the most frequent genetic cause of end-stage renal disease in children and young adults. The genetic mutation has been mapped to chromosome 2q12-q13. In >80% of children with NPH1, the disease is due to a homozygous deletion of the gene. Other patients carry a point mutation in combination with heterozygous deletion. The genes for NPH2, and NPH3 have been mapped to chromosomes 9 and 3 respectively. Sporadic mutations account for about one-sixth of cases.

PATHOGENESIS
The product of the NPH1 gene is a protein of unknown function that contains a src-homology 3 domain called nephrocystin. Because src-homology 3-containing proteins are part of focal adhesion signaling complexes, it has been suggested that the pathogenesis of NPH might be related to abnormalities in signaling processes at the level of cell–matrix or cell–cell interactions. The gene products and the type of genetic mutations for NPH2 and NPH3 are unknown.

CLINICAL HISTORY
Children usually present with polyuria, polydipsia, and nocturnal enuresis reflecting abnormalities in the urinary-concentrating mechanism with a salt-wasting nephropathy present in the majority of patients. The onset of the clinical manifestations is usually after age 2 years but it can occur as early as the first few months of life in children with NPH2. Males and females are equally affected. In up to 30% of patients, anemia precedes the development of renal failure. Similarly, growth retardation that is disproportional to the degree of renal impairment is common. Hypertension is uncommon. Progressive renal failure is insidious, and may remain undetected until end-stage renal failure has developed.

PHYSICAL EXAMINATION
Apart from growth retardation and pallor (anemia), which are out of proportion to the degree of renal insufficiency, the physical examination in patients with juvenile nephronophthisis is unremarkable.

DIFFERENTIAL DIAGNOSIS
Histopathologically, NPH is similar to medullary cystic kidney disease (MCKD). However, MCKD is associated with hyperuricemia and gout and with a much later age of onset of ESRD. While patients with ADPKD or ARPKD usually have significant renal enlargement, with cysts distributed uniformly over the entire organ, in NPH cysts occur primarily at the renal corticomedullary junction, with kidneys typically maintaining a normal size. NPH1 has been reported to occur in association with nystagmus, retinitis pigmentosa and blindness (Senior–Loken syndrome), ocular motor apraxia and retinal degeneration (Cogan syndrome), congenital liver fibrosis, and bone abnormalities, particularly with cone-shaped epiphyses.

INVESTIGATIONS
Urinalysis is normal and proteinuria is usually absent. On renal ultrasound kidneys appear normal or reduced in size, with loss of cortico-medullary differentiation. Thin-section CT scan or MRI examination may detect cysts in the medulla or corticomedullary junction (**192**). As a consequence of the identification of the NPH1 gene, the molecular diagnosis of patients with NPH1 is now possible. The presence of a homozygous deletion of the NPH1 gene is diagnostic for the disease. Heterozygous deletion can be detected by fluorescence *in situ* hybridization, and the specific mutation identified by direct sequencing of all 20 NPH1 exons. If these tests are unavailable, renal biopsy should make the diagnosis.

HISTOLOGY
Histologic findings are similar among the different forms of NPH. Macroscopically, cut sections show a variable number (5–50) of small (up to 2 cm [0.8 in] in diameter), spherical, thin-walled cysts irregularly distributed along the corticomedullary junction. Similar cysts may also occur in the deeper medulla and papillae. No

cysts are detected in up to 25% of cases. Microscopic examination is characterized by disintegration of the tubular basement membrane, tubular atrophy, and interstitial fibrosis, usually without interstitial cell infiltration. Typically, atrophic tubules with thickened basement membranes are clustered next to areas of viable tubules showing dilatation or marked compensatory hypertrophy (**193**). Glomeruli may appear normal or globally sclerosed. On microdissection, cysts appear to originate from cells of the loop of Henle, distal convoluted tubules, and collecting ducts. On electron microscopy, the tubular basement membrane appears irregularly thickened. Some tubules may exhibit an abrupt transition from thick to thin basement membrane, a feature that is characteristic of NPH and rarely seen in other conditions.

PROGNOSIS

NPH commonly results in progressive decline in renal function but the median age for reaching end-stage renal failure varies among the different forms of the disease. Patients with NPH2 reach end-stage renal disease between 1–3 years of age, while the age for NPH1 and NPH3 has been determined to be 13 years and 19 years of age, respectively. The clinical course is similar among members of the same family.

MANAGEMENT

Therapy is supportive. Excessive sodium losses may cause orthostatic hypotension and require sodium supplementation. Patients who reach end-stage renal failure are candidates for dialysis and transplantation.

192 Juvenile nephronophthisis. Renal MRI. Kidneys are relatively normal in size and only 2–3 cysts are clearly visible in each kidney, the largest of which is in the right kidney and measures 1.5 cm (0.6 in) in diameter. The remainder of the cysts are tiny and are localized in the medulla, while others are peripheral near the renal capsule.

193 Juvenile nephronophthisis. Light microscopy showing markedly dilated medullary tubules (H+E x200).

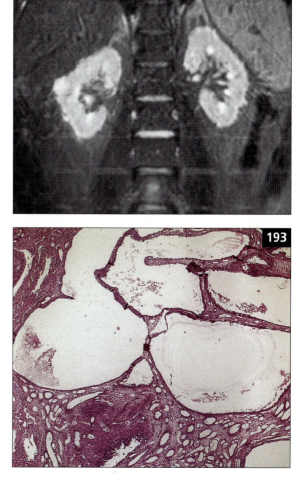

Alport's syndrome

DEFINITION

Alport's syndrome (AS) is an inherited disorder of basement membranes, arising from mutations in type IV collagen. It is characterized by a progressive nephritis manifested by hematuria, frequently associated with a sensorineural hearing loss and ocular abnormalities.

EPIDEMIOLOGY AND ETIOLOGY

The worldwide incidence is approximately 1:10,000, accounting for up to 2% of children with end-stage renal disease. It is seen in all races and geographic areas. In at least 80% of the patients the disease is X-linked. In approximately 5% of cases, an autosomal recessive pattern of inheritance is found. In a few kindreds, the disease follows an autosomal dominant pattern.

PATHOGENESIS

In over half of the patients the disease results from a mutation in the COL4A5 gene on the X chromosome. This gene codes for the $\alpha 5$ chain of type IV collagen $\alpha 5$ (IV). A variety of mutations have been described including deletions, point mutations, and splicing errors. Although the primary molecular defect in AS most commonly involves the $\alpha 5$ (IV) chain, faulty assembly of the $\alpha 3, 4, 5$ heterotrimer produces similar pathologic changes. Failure of normal heterotrimer formation is illustrated by the absence of demonstrable $\alpha 3$ chain of type IV collagen in the glomerular basement membrane in many patients whose genetic defect is in the gene coding for the $\alpha 5(IV)$ chain. In autosomal recessive AS, homozygous or mixed heterozygous mutations of COL4A3 or COL4A4 have been described. Mutations causing autosomal dominant disease have not yet been identified. Concomitant deletions in parts of the COL4A5 and COL4A6 genes occur in familiar forms of esophageal and genital leiomyomatosis.

CLINICAL HISTORY

The basis for diagnosis is the presence of progressive renal disease in a patient with hematuria, sensorineural hearing loss, and family history for AS. Persistent or intermittent microscopic hematuria, with episodes of gross hematuria, is present in virtually all affected males. Hematuria may be exacerbated by exercise or upper respiratory infection. Microscopic hematuria is also common in heterozygous females. Dysmorphic red blood cells and red cells casts are commonly seen. Mild proteinuria is present in most cases and progresses with age, becoming nephrotic in approximately 30% of patients. Hypertension occurs late in the course. Like proteinuria, hypertension is more common in homozygous males than in heterozygous females, but affects both genders equally in patients with the autosomal recessive form. In males, virtually all progress to ESRD, often by age 16–35 years. The disease is usually mild in heterozygous females but some will develop end-stage renal failure, usually after the age of 50 years. The rate of progression to end-stage renal failure is fairly constant among affected males within individual families, but varies significantly from family to family.

High frequency sensorineural hearing loss is present in 30–50% of patients, mainly males. Progressive renal failure does occur in patients without overt hearing loss. Ocular disorders accompany 15–30% of cases. Of the lens abnormalities, anterior lenticonus (**194**) is both the most frequent and specific. Lenticonus is characterized by thinning of the lens capsule resulting in bulging of the lens substance into the anterior chamber, as a result of the defective type IV collagen forming the anterior lens capsule. Progression of the lenticonus results in increasing protrusion of the cone into the anterior chamber and increasing myopia. Anterior lenticonus is diagnosed by the characteristic 'oil droplet in water' effect: a dark disk is seen in the center of the pupillary region on indirect fundoscopy. Other ocular lesions said to be characteristic of AS are macular and mid-peripheral retinal flecks. Macular flecks are round whitish or yellowish granulations surrounding the foveal area. In the periphery of the retina flecks tend to merge and form larger, irregular, circular forms. These changes are not associated with visual impairment.

PHYSICAL EXAMINATION

Overt hearing loss is present in many but not all patients. Anterior lenticonus and retinal flecks are present in a minority of patients.

DIFFERENTIAL DIAGNOSIS

The differential diagnosis involves excluding other causes of microscopic hematuria including renal tumors and structural abnormalities of the urinary tract. Immunofluorescence studies of renal biopsies should rule out IgA nephropathy, membranoproliferative glomerulonephritis, and other immune complex-mediated glomerulonephritis. Once these have been excluded, the main differential diagnosis is with familial glomerular syndromes, in particular thin basement membrane disease.

INVESTIGATIONS

Absence of the $\alpha3$ (IV), $\alpha4$(IV), and $\alpha5$(IV) chains from GBM and distal TBM occur only in patients with AS, and are a diagnostic finding on renal biopsy. Patients with AS frequently lack staining with fluoresceine labelled anti-GBM antibody, and this unique abnormality can be of help in establishing the diagnosis. In families with a previously defined mutation, molecular diagnosis of affected males or gene-carrying females is possible. In families where mutations have not been defined, genetic linkage analysis can determine whether an at-risk individual carries the mutant gene, provided there are at least two other affected members available for testing.

HISTOLOGY (195–197)

On light microscopy lesions are nonspecific. Glomeruli may appear normal or exhibit thickening of capillary walls along with an increase in mesangial matrix. An increased number of fetal glomeruli may be present. Foam cells may be seen in the interstitium. As the disease progresses, progressive glomerular sclerosis and interstitial fibrosis develop. Routine immunofluorescence staining is usually negative. Diagnostic features are usually seen on electron microscopy. At an early stage, thinning of the GBM may be the only visible abnormality, and may suggest thin basement membrane disease. With time, there is thickening of the GBM with splitting of the lamina densa into several irregular layers that may branch and rejoin, giving a characteristic 'basket weave' appearance. The capillary walls show foot processes effacement in variable degrees. Not all patients with AS have these characteristic electron microscopic features.

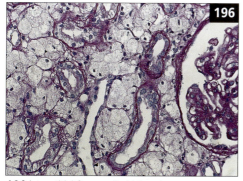

194 Lenticonus.

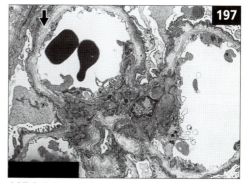

195 Large red cell cast (arrow) within a cortical tubule. Light microscopy (MS x200).

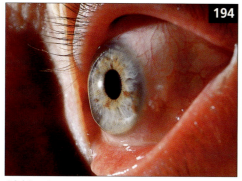

196 Interstitial foam cells. Light microscopy (PAS x250).

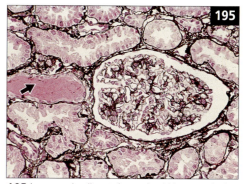

197 Splitting and lamellation of the lamina densa of the basement membrane (arrow). Electron microscopy (x2000).

Alport's syndrome (*continued*)

PROGNOSIS

Virtually all as affected males progress to end-stage renal disease. In heterozygous females, the prognosis is usually benign, with most maintaining preserved renal function long term. Heterozygous females with a history of macroscopic hematuria and nephrotic range proteinuria are likely to develop progressive renal disease. Sensorineural deafness and anterior lenticonus are also predictors of poor outcome in affected women. Patients with autosomal recessive AS, regardless of sex, tend to progress to end-stage renal failure during the second or third decade of life.

MANAGEMENT

There is no specific treatment for AS. Retinal lesions do not affect vision and required no treatment. Lenticonus or cataracts are best treated by removal of the lens with implantation of an intraocular lens. Hearing loss is improved by the use of hearing aids. Tinnitus is generally unresponsive to any form of therapy. Tight control of blood pressure and moderate protein restriction is recommended to retard the progression of renal disease, but the benefit is unproven. Peritoneal dialysis, hemodialysis, and renal transplant are used successfully. Transplanted patients frequently develop anti-GBM antibodies but the risk of developing an anti-GBM crescentic nephritis is lower (5–10%). Alport's patients who have already lost a graft due to anti-GBM-mediated nephritis are at very high risk for recurrence if re-transplanted.

Nail–patella syndrome

DEFINITION

The nail–patella syndrome is a rare (~1:50,000) autosomal dominant disorder characterized by dystrophic nails, absence or hypoplasia of the patella, skeletal deformities, ocular abnormalities, and renal disease.

ETIOLOGY AND PATHOGENESIS

The syndrome has been linked to mutations in the LMX1B gene on chromosome 9. The LMX1B gene appears to be important for normal skeletal and renal development, but the precise mechanisms for the renal effects of the LMX1B mutations remains unknown.

CLINICAL HISTORY

Clinical features include osseous abnormalities, of which the most classical is the absence or hypoplasia of the patella (**198**) (60%), nail changes (80–90%), ocular changes, and renal manifestations (30–40%). The patellae, when present, are subject to recurrent dislocation, and can be associated with effusions and osteoarthritis of the knees. Nail changes are bilateral and symmetric with fingernails, specially the thumbs, more commonly affected than toenails. Nails changes include discoloration, koilonychia, absent or dystrophic nails, V-shaped lunulae, or longitudinal ridges. Ocular abnormalities include abnormal pigmentation of the iris, microcornea, congenital glaucoma, strabismus, or ptosis. Renal involvement is clinically manifested in fewer than half of the patients. Proteinuria and microscopic hematuria are the most common findings. Proteinuria is usually low grade (<3 g/24 h) but it can be nephrotic. Approximately 50% of the patients have impaired ability in concentrating and acidifying the urine. Some patients develop mild hypertension.

PHYSICAL EXAMINATION

Nail dysplasia and patellar aplasia or hypoplasia are essential features for diagnosis. The presence of triangular nail lunulae is a pathognomonic sign. Iliac horns are triangular bony protruberances of the posterior ilium and may be palpable.

DIFFERENTIAL DIAGNOSIS

The typical ultrastructural changes of the GBM of nail–patella syndrome have also been described in a new type of genetic GBM disease named collagen III glomerulopathy.

INVESTIGATIONS

The most common radiologic findings are bilateral iliac horns (**199**) and hypoplasia or absence of the patellae. Humeral and radial abnormalities have also been described including aplasia, hypoplasia, and posterior processes at the distal end of the humerus and hypoplasia of the proximal radial heads. Iliac horns (osseous spurs extending posteriorly from the iliac wings) occur in approximately 80% of patients and are considered pathognomonic for the disease. Radiologic examinations have also detected a number of renal and urinary tract structural abnormalities including dilated calyces and cortical scarring, unilateral renal atrophy, bifid ureter, unilateral hypoplasia and contralateral double kidney, duplication of right pyelocalyceal system, and renal stones.

HISTOLOGY

There are no specific features of nail–patella syndrome on light or immunofluorescence microscopy. On electron microscopy, the glomerular basement membrane is irregularly thickened and contains multiple areas of increased lucency (described as a 'moth-eaten' appearance). These lucent areas can also be seen in the mesangium. Sometimes, the lucent spaces are found to contain coarse fibrillar densities with the appearance and periodicity of collagen, which are better seen after staining the sections with phosphotungstic acid. The fibrils, usually clustered in small collections, have not been found in any other basement membranes except the kidneys. The visceral epithelial foot processes are usually effaced.

PROGNOSIS

Despite proteinuria, renal function is usually preserved in these patients. However, a few patients (10%) will develop progressive renal failure.

MANAGEMENT

There is no specific available treatment for this disease, except for the usual recommendations for management of chronic renal failure, and surgical correction of bone deformities.

198 Absent patella in nail–patella syndrome.

199 Pelvis X-ray showing bilateral iliac horns.

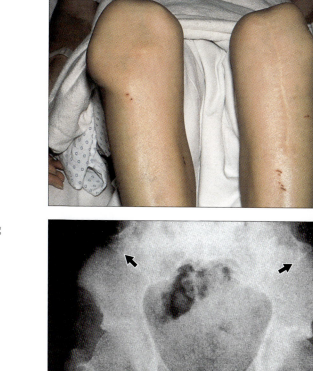

Congenital nephrotic syndrome

DEFINITION
Congenital nephrotic syndrome (CNS) is defined as the presence of nephrotic syndrome at the time of birth or within the first 3 months of life.

EPIDEMIOLOGY AND ETIOLOGY
CNS can occur as a manifestation of a number of disorders (*Table 10*). The 'classic' or Finnish type is the most common and best known of all the types of CNS. It is inherited as an autosomal recessive trait, with an incidence of 1:8000 births in Finland. The incidence is significantly lower in other countries. The disease is caused by mutation on a novel 29-exon gene (the NPHS1 gene) localized to chromosome 19q13.1, coding for a transmembrane 1241 amino acid protein of the immunoglobulin superfamily termed nephrin. The two most common mutations in the NPHS1 gene have been named Fin-major and Fin-minor. The Fin-major is a frameshift mutation resulting in a truncated protein of only 90 amino acids. Fin-minor mutation is a nonsense mutation leading to a truncated 1109-residue protein. Sixty-five per cent of the Finnish patients have been found to be homozygous for the Fin-major mutation, while 8% are homozygous for Fin-minor. A number of other mutations, including insertions, deletions, nonsense and missense mutations have been described in non-Finnish patients.

Table 10 Causes of congenital nephrotic syndrome
<ul><li>'Classic' or Finnish type</li><li>Diffuse mesangial sclerosis (DMS)</li><li>Idiopathic</li><li>Denys–Drash syndrome (DMS, male pseudohermaphroditism, and Wilms tumor)</li><li>Galloway–Mowat syndrome (DMS, microcephaly, gyral abnormalities, and developmental delay)</li><li>Idiopathic focal and segmental glomerulosclerosis (FSGS)</li><li>Genetic disorders</li><li>Mucopolysaccharidosis</li><li>Infantile sialic acid storage</li><li>Carbohydrate-deficient-glycoprotein syndrome</li><li>Nail–patella syndrome</li><li>Lowe's syndrome</li><li>Congenital infections</li><li>Syphilis</li><li>Cytomegalovirus</li><li>Toxoplasmosis</li><li>Mercury</li><li>Infantile systemic lupus erythematosus</li></ul>

PATHOGENESIS
Nephrin is produced by glomerular podocytes and it is localized at the slit diaphragm. Electron microscopy studies of kidney samples obtained from patients with Fin-major and Fin-minor mutations show abnormalities of the slit diaphragm. This suggests that nephrin is an important component of the slit diaphragm and plays a crucial role in maintaining glomerular permselectivity. Recent studies suggest that nephrin is also involved in the development of proteinuria in other glomerular disease.

CLINICAL HISTORY
The classic findings in CNS of the Finnish type include prematurity, large placenta, and proteinuria, which already begins *in utero*. Due to the large placenta, difficulties at delivery are common, including postural deformities and malpresentation. Progressive ascites refractory to diuretics develops and interferes with feeding, resulting in severe growth failure and developmental delay. Umbilical hernias are common.

Due to the severity of the nephrotic syndrome, infections are common, and account for up to one-third of the overall mortality. Thromboembolic complications are also frequent.

PHYSICAL EXAMINATION
Edema and abdominal distension, mainly caused by ascites, is present at birth in 25% of cases. These signs develop in an additional 25% of cases during the first week of life, and full-blown nephrotic syndrome is manifested in all patients by the age of 3 months. With time, reduced subcutaneous tissue and muscular wasting is clearly visible.

DIFFERENTIAL DIAGNOSIS
The main differential diagnosis is with diffuse mesangial sclerosis (DMS) and FSGS. In patients with DMS, nephrotic syndrome usually manifests after the second month of life. Progression to end-stage renal failure with hypertension by the age of 2 years is usual. The pathology may be associated with male pseudohermaphroditism (Denys–Drash

syndrome) and microcephaly (Galloway–Mowat syndrome). FSGS is the most common histopathologic finding in children with steroid-resistant nephrotic syndrome. In some cases, proteinuria may be present at birth. A heterogeneous group of disorders accounts for the rest of cases of CNS (*Table 10*).

INVESTIGATIONS

Nephrotic range proteinuria and low serum albumin levels are usually present immediately after birth. Microscopic hematuria and leukocyturia are also common. Serum creatinine and glomerular filtration rate are usually within normal limits during the first 3 months of life but renal function decreases slowly thereafter. Serum albumin levels are significantly reduced, with a mean value <0.5 g/dl (5 g/l). Raised α-fetoprotein levels are present in the amniotic fluid, and sometimes in the maternal plasma, which may indicate the development of CNS *in utero*.

HISTOLOGY

Histopathologic examination shows mesangial hypercellularity, hyper lobulated capillary tufts, and some scarring. Proximal and distal tubuli may show microcystic dilatation. Scattered inflammation and fibrosis can be observed in the interstitium. Electron microscopy shows glomerular podocyte fusion (**200**). Immunohistochemistry studies can confirm the absence of nephrin on the podocyte surface. Later, diffuse mesangial sclerosis and significant interstitial fibrosis are present in the cortex.

PROGNOSIS

Without active treatment, prognosis is poor. Before the end of their first year 75% of children with Finnish type CNS have died; only 3% have lived to the age of 2 years; and none has reach 4 years of age. With transplantation, there may be a remarkable catch-up growth and developmental progress.

MANAGEMENT

Current treatment of children with CNS includes active protein and nutritional support, including albumin and immunoglobulin infusion, high-protein low-salt diet, diuretics, and antibiotic prophylaxis. During the nephrotic state, prophylactic anticoagulation is recommended to reduce the risk of thromboembolic complications. Some children will require thyroid hormone replacement therapy. Classic CNS (Finnish type) patients usually do not respond to the use of ACE inhibitors or indomethacin, although anecdotal cases have been reported. Similarly, corticosteroids and immunosuppressive drugs are also ineffective. Conservative therapy should be followed with bilateral nephrectomy and dialysis, prior to undergoing renal transplantation. Renal replacement therapy is effectively achieved with peritoneal dialysis. Several months on this treatment are required in order to allow the patient to recover from the severity of the nephrotic syndrome, and renal transplantation is most commonly delayed until the child reaches 8–9 kg (18–20 lb) of body weight (usually in the second or third year of life).

200 Congenital Finnish nephrosis. Electron microscopy showing diffuse effacement of visceral epithelial foot processes with microvillous transformation. Visceral epithelial cells are vacuolated (×3400).

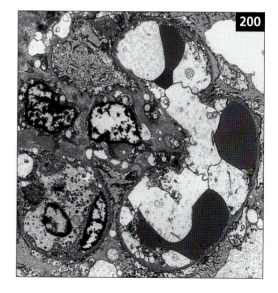

Fabry disease (Anderson–Fabry disease, angiokeratoma corporis diffusum)

DEFINITION
Fabry disease is the clinical and pathologic manifestations of an inborn error of glycosphingolipid metabolism, secondary to deficiency of the lysosomal enzyme alpha-galactosidase A (αGalA).

EPIDEMIOLOGY AND ETIOLOGY
Fabry disease is a rare (1:40,000) X-linked disorder linked to mutations in the gene encoding for αGalA, which is located on chromosome X, Xq22>q24. The disease is more common in whites, but it has been reported in other races. It characteristically affects males. Heterozygous females may have mild manifestations of the disease but severe Fabry disease has been documented in females who have inactivation of the normal αGalA allele. The specific mutations vary between individuals and accounts for the variable clinical expression of the enzymatic defect.

PATHOGENESIS
The lysosomal enzyme αGalA is responsible for the hydrolysis of ceramide to sphingosine and free fatty acid. Deficiency of αGalA results in intracellular accumulation of neutral glycosphingolipids, predominantly ceramide trihexoside, in tissues throughout the body. Blood vessel cells, renal epithelium, corneal epithelium, myocardium, and ganglion cells of the autonomic nervous system are primarily affected, but glycosphingolipid accumulation occurs in virtually every organ of the body. With time, this process leads to a multisystem dysfunction. Because of the accumulation of B-specific glycosphingolipids, patients with blood types B and AB have earlier and more severe clinical presentations.

CLINICAL HISTORY AND PHYSICAL EXAMINATION
Fabry disease is a multisystem disorder affecting the skin, heart, peripheral and central nervous systems, and the kidneys. Renal involvement is common and is manifested by hematuria and proteinuria (<3 g/24 h) beginning in the third decade of life, with gradual progression to end-stage renal failure in the fourth or fifth decades. Skin involvement is characterized by the presence of angiokeratomas (**201**) which appear as red-purple macules or papules typically located in the lower abdomen, buttocks, hips, genitalia, or upper thighs. The number of lesions varies from 20–40, but they may be few or absent. Size can also vary from a few microns to several millimeters. On histology, angiokeratoma consists of small upper dermal dilated veins, covered by a hyperkeratotic epidermis. Other skin manifestations include palmar erythema, telangiectasias and subungual splinter hemorrhages. Neurologic compromise is characterized by peripheral and autonomic neuropathy, and cerebrovascular complications. Autonomic neuropathy is manifested by acral paresthesias, which are exacerbated by fever or exercise, hypohydrosis, impaired pupillary constriction, and abnormal intestinal motility. Temperature sensation may be impaired reflecting peripheral nerve involvement.

Cerebrovascular disease can present as seizures, transient ischemic attacks, or completed strokes. The vertebrobasilar circulation is most frequently affected and disease can be manifested by vertigo, nausea, vomiting, nystagmus, diplopia, and ataxia. Repeated strokes can lead to significant memory loss or dementia. Corneal opacities are seen in virtually all patients and in the majority of heterozygous carriers. By slit-lamp examination, they appear as whorls of whitish discoloration that radiate from the center to the periphery of the cornea. Other ocular findings include posterior capsular cataracts, retina and eyelid edema, and retinal and conjunctival telangiectasias. Heart involvement can be manifested by development of angina, myocardial infarction, or congestive heart failure. Finally, generalized lymphadenopathy, hepatosplenomegaly, myopathy, and aseptic necrosis of the femoral and humeral heads have been described to occur in some patients.

DIFFERENTIAL DIAGNOSIS
Fabry disease should be considered in the differential diagnosis of stroke or renal disease of unknown etiology, or fever, pain, and skin lesions of unknown origin. Potential misdiagnoses include rheumatoid or juvenile arthritis, rheumatic fever, SLE, and multiple sclerosis (stroke-like events).

INVESTIGATIONS
The diagnosis can be confirmed by demonstrating reduced activity of αGalA in peripheral blood leukocytes. In homozygote males there is almost no enzyme activity. Female heterozygotes have enzyme levels that are intermediate between normal and homozygote patients. Carriers for the disease can be identified by measuring ceramide digalactoside and trihexoside levels in the urine. During childhood, birefringent lipid globules with

a characteristic 'Maltese cross' shape can be observed in the urine by polarization microscopy.

HISTOLOGY

The glomerular visceral epithelial cell is the primary site of glycosphingolipid accumulation. On light microscopy these cells appear enlarged and vacuolated. The vacuoles, which represent lipid material that has been extracted during processing, are small, uniformly distributed, and have a foamy or 'honeycomb' appearance. Similar vacuolated cells are also present in epithelial cells of distal convoluted tubules and loop of Henle, but are rarely seen in the mesangium or proximal tubules. Extensive vacuolation is also seen in the arterial vessels. Progressive renal involvement results in the development of segmental and global glomerulosclerosis. Immunofluorescence microscopy is typically negative, except for areas of advanced sclerosis where IgM and complement may be present. On electron microscopy cellular inclusions are localized almost entirely within lysosomes (202). The inclusions are present in all cells, regardless of the light microscopy features, and vary in size, shape, number, and location, according to the different cells. They are typically round and are composed of concentric layers of dense material separated by clear spaces giving an 'onion skin' appearance ('myelin figures'), or may have an ovoid shape with the dense layers arranged in parallel ('zebra bodies'). Inclusions are also seen in heterozygous females although to a lesser degree.

PROGNOSIS

The survival rate for patients on dialysis is approximately 40% at 5 years. Neurologic and cardiovascular complications account for the increased mortality in these patients.

MANAGEMENT

Recombinant α-galactosidase A is available as infusion therapy. It has been shown to stabilize glomerular filtration rate, reduce pain, improve cardiac conduction, and reverse cardiomyopathy. Patients with end-stage renal failure can be treated by dialysis, or by renal transplantation. Renal transplantation does not affect the extrarenal manifestations.

201 Angiokeratoma located on the umbilicus.

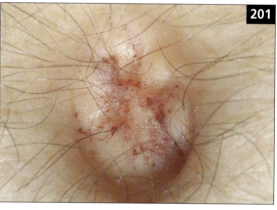

202 Electron microscopy demonstrating 'myelin figures' (arrow) within the lysosomes in visceral epithelial and endothelial cells (×8000).

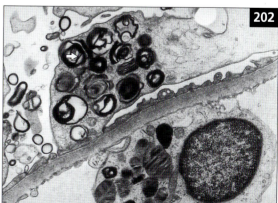

Von Hippel–Lindau disease

DEFINITION

Von Hippel–Lindau (VHL) disease is an autosomal dominant cancer syndrome characterized by the presence of benign and malignant tumors. Hallmark lesions include retinal angiomas, hemangioblastomas of the central nervous system, renal cell carcinomas, and pheochromocytomas.

EPIDEMIOLOGY AND ETIOLOGY

The disease occurs in all ethnic groups and affects both sexes equally. It has an estimated incidence of approximately 1:40,000 births. Diagnosis is usually made in the third or fourth decade but increases with age. Penetrance has been estimated at 80–90% by age 65 years, although expression is highly variable. All patients with this disease harbor a germ line mutation of the VHL gene located on chromosome 3p25. Tumor development is linked to loss or inactivation of the remaining wild-type VHL allele.

PATHOGENESIS

The product of the VHL gene, pVHL, is important in the regulation of a transcription factor called hypoxia-inducible factor (HIF). In the presence of oxygen, pVHL polyubiquitinates HIFα subunits which targets HIF for proteosomal degradation. In the absence of pVHL, HIFα subunits cannot be degraded and consequently will overstimulate HIF target genes. Among these are genes implicated in angiogenesis, such as VEGF (vascular endothelial growth factor) and PDGF-B (platelet-derived growth factor B chain). Thus, the vascular nature of VHL-associated tumors is explained by the overproduction of angiogenic factors encoded by HIF-stimulated genes. In this sense, the VHL gene behaves as a tumor suppressor gene.

CLINICAL HISTORY

There are several characteristic features of VHL. The renal lesions in VHL include both cysts and carcinomas (**203**). Renal cysts are present in over half of the patient. They may be solitary, but most frequently are bilateral and multiple and occasionally can mimic autosomal dominant polycystic kidney disease (ADPKD). Unlike ADPKD, renal cysts in VHL rarely cause hypertension or progressive renal failure. In patients with VHL there is an increased incidence of renal cell carcinomas. Tumors are often bilateral. Thirty to fifty percent of patients with symptomatic renal carcinoma will have metastatic disease. In patients with VHL, pheochromocytomas differ from those in sporadic cases in that they occur in younger patients, and are often bilateral, multiple, and extra-adrenal. They are often asymptomatic and rarely metastasize. Patients with VHL and pheochromocytomas cluster in families. Angiomatous or cystic lesions may also occur in the pancreas and the epididymis.

Central nervous system hemangioblastomas occur more frequently in the cerebellum followed by the spine and the brain stem (**204, 205**). Tumors are often multiple and occur at a younger age than in patients with sporadic cases. The hemangioblastomas are benign, but they may produce symptoms, including nausea, vomiting, headache, and vertigo, depending on their number, size, and site. In over 50% of the patients angiomas (hemangioblastomas) are present in the retina (**206**). Tumors are often multiple, bilateral, and recurrent. The most serious complications are retinal hemorrhage and retinal detachment that may lead to blindness.

PHYSICAL EXAMINATION

Signs of central nervous system involvement include papilledema, ataxia, slurred speech, and nystagmus. Retinal angiomas appear as reddish spherical tumors of variable size with a dilated feeding artery and a draining vein.

DIFFERENTIAL DIAGNOSIS

The differential diagnosis of renal lesions in VHL includes ADPKD and tuberous sclerosis complex (TSC). Patients with VHL are usually normotensive, have normal renal function, and have fewer and smaller renal cysts than patients with ADPKD. Renal cell carcinomas are uncommon in ADPKD. Liver cysts are common in ADPKD but are rarely seen in VHL. In both TSC and VHL multiple renal cysts and tumors occur. However, renal tumors in TSC are usually angiomyolipomas and the extrarenal manifestations help to differentiate TSC from VHL.

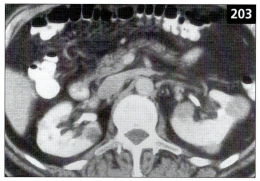

203 CT scan showing bilateral solid and cystic renal masses.

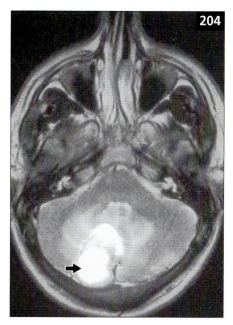

204 MRI showing cerebellar hemangioblastoma (arrow).

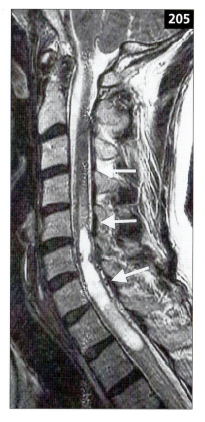

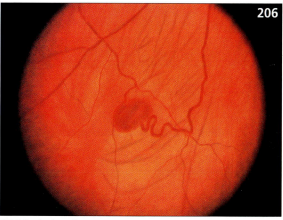

206 Retinal angioma.

205 T2-MRI sagittal image of the cervical spine showing a partially cystic intramedullary neoplasm expanding the spinal cord. Note the dilated pial vascularity (arrows).

Von Hippel–Lindau disease (*continued*)

INVESTIGATIONS

Detection of central nervous system hemangioblastomas has improved substantially with the use of gadolinium-enhanced magnetic resonance imaging. Genetic testing can be used to identify carriers of VHL gene mutations. Mutations can be detected in over 80% of families with VHL. In the remaining patients, genetic linkage analysis can help to identify individuals carrying a mutant VHL gene provided that there are at least two other affected members available for testing.

HISTOLOGY

Microscopically, kidneys from patients with VHL may contain numerous small neoplasms. Cysts are lined by a flattened, nondescriptive or cuboidal clear cell epithelium that may appear as focal nodular hyperplasia, or intracystic renal cell carcinomas. In patients with renal cell tumors, the predominant histologic finding is a clear cell carcinoma.

PROGNOSIS

The development of multiple central nervous system tumors is still a major problem, and central nervous system involvement is an important cause of morbidity and mortality in these patients. Patients with VHL have a lifetime risk >70% for developing a renal cell carcinoma, and these tumors cause death in up to 50% of VHL patients. In patients with VHL, early cancer screening beginning in childhood with ophthalmoscopy and magnetic resonance imaging of brain, spine, and abdomen, has a direct beneficial impact on the long-term prognosis.

MANAGEMENT

In patients who develop central nervous system symptoms secondary to a tumor-mass effect, surgical resection of hemangioblastomas often provides excellent results. Regular ophthalmologic examinations are an essential component of the preventive screening. Retinal angiomas can be treated by laser and cryotherapy. Early intervention is recommended to ensure preservation of vision. Annual surveillance with CT, ultrasonography, or both is indicated for early detection of renal cell carcinomas. Treatment of solid lesions is by parenchymal-sparing surgery whenever possible, in order to avoid or delay the need for dialysis or transplantation. Repeated surgical intervention is usually required as tumors continue to develop. Symptomatic pheochromocytomas must be removed surgically. It is important to attempt to localize extra-adrenal tumors pre-operatively in order to prevent life-threatening complications during surgery, because of unexpected tumor manipulation. Because of the increased risk of cancer, family screening is imperative, including analysis of mutations. Patients who did not inherit the mutant gene do not need further evaluation. Patients who are carriers for a VHL mutation or at-risk individuals in whom the presence of a mutation cannot be determined need periodic screening for occult disease manifestation.

Primary hyperoxalurias (PH)

DEFINITION

PHs are autosomal recessive disorders characterized by metabolic overproduction of oxalate resulting in urolithiasis, nephrocalcinosis, and accumulation of insoluble oxalate throughout the body.

EPIDEMIOLOGY AND ETIOLOGY

There are two types of PH that result from different enzymatic defects in the hepatic glyoxalate pathway. In type I PH the defective enzyme is alanine glyoxylate aminotransferase (AGT). In humans the AGT gene is encoded on chromosome 2q36-37. Differences in the type of mutation results in a varied pattern in AGT enzyme expression: total absence (~30% of patients), presence of an inactive enzyme (~25%), or selective mistargeting of the enzyme from peroxisomes to the mitochondria (~40%). PHs are rare disorders. Type I PH occurs in ~ 1:120,000 live births, but incidence is much more frequent when parental consanguinity is present. Type II PH is an even rarer disorder that is due to deficiency of hepatic hydroxypyruvate reductase. The gene encoding for this enzyme is localized on chromosome 9 and specific mutations have been described in a small number of patients.

PATHOGENESIS

Oxalate is a poorly soluble end product of metabolism. In humans, oxalate excretion is mainly renal, although there is increasing evidence that the gastrointestinal tract, mainly the colon, also plays a role. Approximately 80–90% of the daily oxalate excreted in the urine is produced endogenously, with only 10–20% being of dietary origin. Dietary oxalate originates mainly from fruits and vegetables. Absorption occurs throughout the entire intestine, but mostly in the small bowel. Total colectomy does not appear to alter oxalate absorption, but increased colonic absorption occurs in patients with enteric hyperoxaluria. Formation of oxalate occurs in the liver through a partially understood metabolic pathway. Hepatic peroxisomal AGT and hydroxypyruvate reductase are key enzymes in this pathway. AGT is needed for converting glyoxylate to glycine, thus diverting glyoxylate from being oxidized to oxalate. Pyridoxine is a co-factor in the AGT pathway. In type II, deficiency in hydroxypyruvate reductase results in failure of glyoxalate reduction to glycolate, but the cause of increased oxalate production is unclear. In the kidney, oxalate is freely filtered by the glomerulus and then undergoes a complex absorption and secretion process. The upper limit for renal excretion is approximately 40 mg/24 h. Excessive ingestion of oxalate in the diet can result in increased urinary oxalate, but rarely exceeds 60 mg/24 h. In PH, however, urinary oxalate levels may range from 80–300 mg/24 h. Within the kidney, crystal deposition results in intratubular obstruction. Rupture of the tubular epithelial allows oxalate to migrate to the interstitium where it triggers a severe inflammatory response. With time, the chronic interstitial process will result in progressive loss of renal function.

CLINICAL HISTORY AND PHYSICAL EXAMINATION

In either, type I or II PH, the disease is most often manifested during the first or second decade of life with symptoms related to the urinary tract: loin pain, hematuria, urinary tract infections, or passage of a renal stone. In some patients, the disease may remain unrecognized until well into adulthood. Some patients may present with end-stage renal failure without a preceding history of urolithiasis. In patients with preserved renal function, plasma oxalate levels remain close to normal, with the main clinical problem being urolithiasis. With time, the increased renal deposition of oxalate and stone formation will result in variable degrees of obstruction, progressive renal interstitial fibrosis, and renal failure. Once glomerular filtration rate falls below 30 ml/min, continued overproduction of oxalate by the liver along with reduced renal oxalate excretion results in increasing oxalate deposition in many organs. The major compartment of the insoluble oxalate pool is bone, and therefore bone disease is the most disabling complication of oxalosis. Along with the skeleton, systemic involvement includes: the cardiovascular system (cardiomyopathy, conduction defects, disseminated vascular occlusive lesions), nerves (peripheral neuropathy, mononeuritis multiplex), joints (synovitis), skin (calcinosis, livedo reticularis), soft tissues, liver, and retina.

Primary hyperoxalurias (PH) (*continued*)

DIFFERENTIAL DIAGNOSIS

Other causes of hyperoxaluria include intestinal (hyperabsorptive) hyperoxaluria, enteric hyperabsorption (e.g. ileal resection, pancreatic insufficiency, Crohn's disease, malabsorption), excessive dietary ingestion of substances containing oxalic acid (e.g. cocoa, tea, spinach, nuts), or poisoning (e.g. ethylene glycol). High plasma oxalate levels also occur in patients with chronic renal failure due to other causes.

INVESTIGATIONS

The diagnosis of a type I PH is strongly suggested in a patient with a marked increase in urinary oxalate excretion (usually >100 mg/24 h) and an elevated urine glycolate, and these findings may be sufficient to establish the diagnosis in patients with typical clinical features. However, up to 25% of patients with type I PH will have urinary glycolate levels within the normal range, and may require a liver biopsy for AGT analysis to confirm the diagnosis. Nephrocalcinosis, best demonstrated by ultrasound, is present on plain abdominal radiograph in patients with advanced stages of the disease (**207**). Linkage studies or direct detection of mutation are useful diagnostic tools but, at present, <50% of cases can be diagnosed by DNA testing. In patients with chronic renal failure, urinary oxalate and glycolate excretion may be normal. In this situation, plasma oxalate and plasma glycolate will be markedly elevated. Interpretation of plasma oxalate levels in patients on dialysis is difficult because most patients with end-stage renal failure from other causes will have elevated plasma oxalate levels. In patients with type II PH, the diagnosis is suggested by the findings of marked urinary oxalate, urine glycerate, and normal urine glycolate.

HISTOLOGY

Macroscopically, calculi are commonly seen within the pelvis and calyceal system. Microscopically, the hallmark of the renal disease is the presence of abundant calcium oxalate deposits within the nephron associated with chronic tubulointerstitial nephritis (**208**). The glomeruli may appear normal or focally sclerosed. Interstitial lesions include giant cell formation, lymphocytic infiltration, and interstitial fibrosis. Crystals vary in shape from round to elongate, often fan-shaped, and are birefringent.

PROGNOSIS

PH is associated with serious morbidity and mortality. Without aggressive treatment, including transplantation, the majority of patients will die before the third decade of life. The earlier the diagnosis, the better the chance of improving the prognosis and quality of life in patients. Aggressive conservative treatment and pre-emptive transplantation have significantly improved the long-term outcome.

MANAGEMENT

The main goal of treatment is to increase oxalate solubility and decrease production. A high urinary output is crucial and patients are required to drink a fluid load large enough to maintain a urinary volume of at least 3 l/24 h. In patients with type I PH, treatment with pyridoxine (vitamin B6) may reduce oxalate production to normal or near normal in up to 30% of cases. Urine alkalinization (target pH >6.5) will increase the solubility of calcium and oxalate. Magnesium also inhibits urinary stone formation and can be given orally either as magnesium gluconate or as magnesium oxide. Orthophosphate is also effective in decreasing calcium oxalate supersaturation and inhibiting urinary calcium precipitation and can be used safely in patients with preserved renal function (clearance >30 ml/min). Low oxalate diet is of limited value in patients with PH.

To remove sufficient oxalate, daily hemodialysis, with 6–8 hours per session, is required. The only curative treatment is liver transplantation to replace the defective liver enzyme. In selected patients, isolated liver transplant is the therapy of choice and should be performed before chronic renal failure onset. Combined kidney and liver transplantation is indicated for patients with advanced renal failure. Following combined kidney and liver transplant, care should be taken to protect the kidney against the damage that can be induced by the heavy oxalate load that results from the rapid mobilization of oxalate accumulated in the tissues.

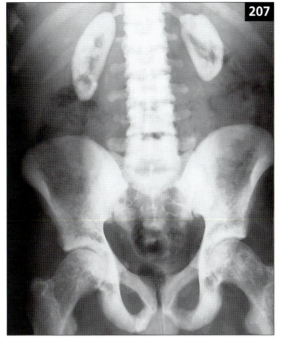

207 Plain abdominal radiograph showing dense nephrocalcinosis and characteristic bone changes in a patient with primary hyperoxaluria and end-stage renal failure.

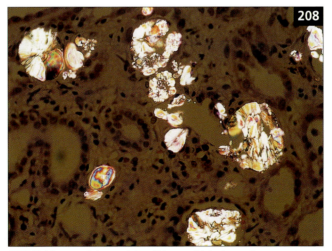

208 Calcium oxalate crystals within renal tubules under cross-polarized light. Light microscopy (H+E x250).

Cystinosis

DEFINITION
Cystinosis is a metabolic disease characterized by excessive intracellular accumulation, particularly in lysosomes, of the amino acid cystine.

EPIDEMIOLOGY AND ETIOLOGY
The disease is inherited as an autosomal recessive trait. It has an estimated incidence of 1:200,000 live births. The cause is a defect in a gene mapped to chromosome 17p13, coding for an integral lysosomal membrane protein, cystostatin, responsible for transporting cystine out of the lysosome. The disease is more common in Caucasians but other races are affected.

PATHOGENESIS
In cystinosis, the defect in the lysosome transporter for cystine results in cystinotic cells accumulating 50–100 times the normal cystine values. The low solubility of cystine results in crystal formation within lysosomes. How crystal formation results in cellular injury is unclear. It has been postulated that accumulated intracellular cystine may interact with sulphydryl groups disrupting sulphydryl-dependent enzyme systems.

CLINICAL HISTORY AND PHYSICAL EXAMINATION
Three different clinical forms of cystinosis can be distinguished based on the clinical course and the intracellular cystine content: infantile (or nephropathic) cystinosis, adolescent or late-onset cystinosis, and benign or adult cystinosis. Infantile cystinosis is the most common form. The disease is usually diagnosed between 6 and 18 months of age with symptoms of excessive thirst and urination, failure to thrive, rickets (**209**), and frequent episodes of dehydration. These findings are a result of a Fanconi syndrome. Subtle abnormalities of tubular function can be demonstrated earlier in families with other affected children, but they are not present at birth. Children with cystinosis also develop cystine crystals in the cornea (after the first year of life) (**210**). Photophobia is common and is progressive, but visual impairment and blindness are rare. A few patients have developed renal calculi. Without specific treatment, patients develop end-stage renal failure by late childhood (7–10 years of age). Late complications include muscle wasting, difficulty swallowing, diabetes,

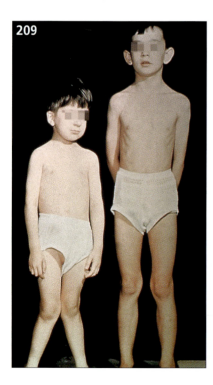

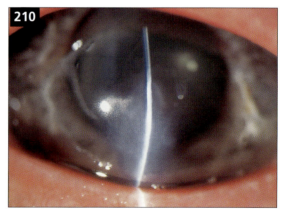

210 Corneal cystine crystals.

209 A patient with cystinosis (left) is shown alongside a normal boy of the same age. The renal rickets is secondary to the amino acid loss and defective calcium and phosphate reabsorption.

hypothyroidism, hepatomegaly and spleno-megaly, corneal ulcerations, and decreased visual acuity. In patients with benign or adult cystino-sis, intracellular cystine levels are mildly elevated with cystine crystals present in the cornea and bone marrow only. These patients do not develop renal failure. Patients with the ado-lescent form have intracellular cystine levels that are intermediate between those of the infantile and adult forms.

DIFFERENTIAL DIAGNOSIS

Childhood Fanconi syndrome is most com-monly the result of cystinosis. Other causes of Fanconi syndrome include nephrotoxicity from heavy metals (cadmium, lead) and systemic diseases (myeloma, fructose intolerance, galac-tosemia, and Wilson disease).

INVESTIGATIONS

The diagnosis is based on detecting increased intracellular cystine levels in white blood cells or skin fibroblasts. Normal cells contain <0.3 nmol half cystine/mg protein. Carriers of cystinosis have levels between 0.3 and 1.0 nmol half cystine/mg protein while those affected with cystinosis have levels above this range. Prenatal diagnosis can be made by measuring cystine levels in cells obtained by chorionic villus sampling or amniocentesis in families where there is a known risk of cystinosis. Chorionic villus sampling is performed at 8–9 weeks of gestation; amniocentesis can be performed at 14–16 weeks of gestation.

HISTOLOGY

Histologic findings vary with the stage of the disease. Early findings include cystine crystal deposition in tubular epithelial and interstitial cells, but rarely in glomerular epithelial cells (211). By nephron microdissection, a shorten-ing and swan-neck deformity of the initial portion of the proximal tubules has been described, but this finding is not specific for cystinosis. Later in the disease, there is progres-sive interstitial fibrosis, periglomerular fibrosis, and glomerulosclerosis. Abundant deposition of small, brick-shaped, hexagonal, or needle-shaped birefringent crystals is found with multi-nucleated, giant cell formation in the glomeruli visceral epithelium and atrophic proximal tubules. On electron microscopy, crystalline inclusions can be seen inside the cells.

PROGNOSIS

The renal prognosis has improved with cys-teamine treatment. It remains to be determined whether children treated with cysteamine from infancy will be spared from the other compli-cations of cystinosis.

MANAGEMENT

Treatment of the Fanconi syndrome involves replacement of the urinary losses of water, electrolytes, bicarbonate, and minerals. Some patients also need vitamin D therapy. The use of indomethacin may be of benefit in patients with severe polyuria. Cysteamine treatment has proven effective in reducing cystine accumu-lation within the cells and delaying the decline in GFR, especially if started earlier in the course of the disease. Cysteamine is easily transported inside lysosomes where it combines with cystine, forming cysteine and a mixed disulfide cys-teamine–cysteine compound. Both cysteine and the disulfide compound exit the lysosome via transport mechanisms other than the cystine carrier. Cysteamine also improves the growth of cystinosis children, although it does not lessen the severity of the Fanconi syndrome. Treat-ment should be started as soon as the diagnosis is made with low doses of cysteamine bitartrate. Side-effects of cysteamine therapy include nausea, vomiting, and a foul odor and taste. Leukocyte cysteine levels should be checked every 3–4 months and therapy adjusted to maintaining cysteine levels below 1.0 nmol half cystine/mg protein. Renal transplantation is the treatment of choice for patients who develop end-stage renal failure, as the disease does not recur in the allograft. Renal transplantation does not improve the extrarenal manifestations of cystinosis.

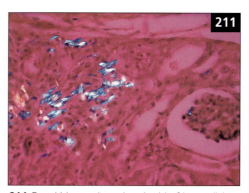

211 Renal biopsy viewed under birefringent light showing interstitial cystine crystals (×100).

Tuberous sclerosis complex (TSC)

DEFINITION
TSC is an autosomal dominant disorder in which patients develop hamartomatous lesions in many different organs, most commonly in the brain, heart, kidney, and skin.

EPIDEMIOLOGY AND ETIOLOGY
TSC has an estimated prevalence of 1:10,000. It affects both sexes equally, with no race predilection. Mean age at diagnosis is the third decade. The disease is caused by mutations in two different genes, which are located on chromosomes 9q32p34 (TSC1) and 16p13 (TSC2). There is a high frequency of spontaneous mutations with sporadic forms accounting for approximately 60% of newly diagnosed cases. There is great variability in the disease penetrance and clinical presentation, with only 50% of patients having a positive family history.

PATHOGENESIS
Both TSC1 and TSC2 genes have been identified and sequenced. The protein product of TSC1 is called hamartin. TSC2 produces a 5.5kb transcript whose protein has been named tuberin. Both are tumor suppressor genes involved in regulation of cell growth and differentiation. The precise mechanism of hamartomatous growth is not completely understood.

CLINICAL HISTORY AND PHYSICAL EXAMINATION
In this disease, multiple hamartomatous tumors develop in multiple organs, including the skin (**212–214**), brain, retina (**215**), liver, bone, heart, lung, and kidney. The most common clinical manifestations are related to the skin and central nervous system. Skin manifestations include facial angiofibromas (adenoma seb-

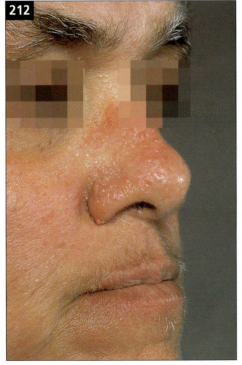

212 Facial angiofibroma.

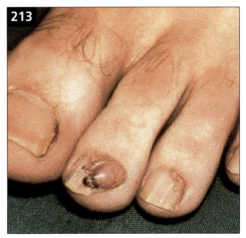

213 Periungual fibroma.

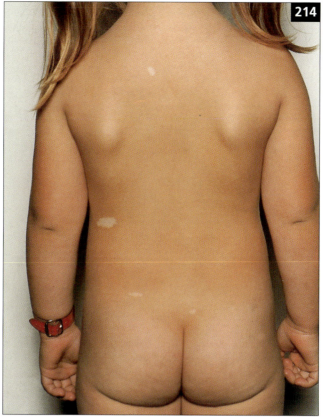

214 Hypomelanotic macule.

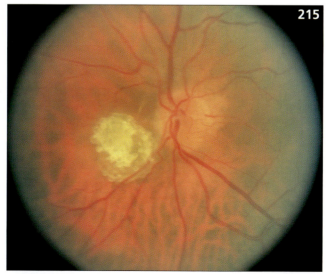

215 Retinal hamartoma.

Tuberous sclerosis complex (TSC) (*continued*)

aceum), ungual fibromas (Koenen tumors), hypomelanotic macules (ash-leaf spots), and shagreen patches. Central nervous system involvement is manifested by the development of seizures and mental retardation. Many patients are neurologically normal despite radiographic evidence of typical brain lesions such as subependymal calcifications (**216**). Renal involvement occurs frequently in TSC (**217, 218**). It is manifested by the presence of hypertension, angiomyolipomas, and renal cysts.

Angiomyolipomas are the main form of hamartomas in TSC. They are multiple and usually bilateral. An important aspect of angiomyolipomas is their potential for bleeding that can be manifested as macroscopic hematuria or retroperitoneal hemorrhage. Bilateral renal angiomyolipomas may also cause chronic renal failure. Angiomyolipomas are larger in females than in males, suggesting a sex hormone effect. Cysts are usually numerous and small, but large cysts do occur and may be confused with polycystic kidney disease. Cysts and angiomyolipomas may be present in combination or only one type may be present. The CT finding of angiomyolipomas and cysts occurring together is strongly suggestive of TSC. An association with renal carcinomas has also been described. Carcinomas are frequently bilateral. Some malignant tumors are now recognized as malignant epithelioid angiomyolipomas.

The diagnosis is based on clinical, radiologic, and biopsy findings. The disease however presents great phenotypic variability with size, number, and location of lesions differing significantly among patients, even in members of the same family. Specific clinical criteria have been defined for the diagnosis of TSC (*Table 11*).

DIFFERENTIAL DIAGNOSIS

Renal cysts and angiomyolipomas can occur as sporadic lesions in individuals not affected by TSC. Sometimes, renal imaging can mimic autosomal dominant polycystic kidney disease. The TSC2 gene is positioned next to the PKD1 gene, and a contiguous TSC2/PKD1 gene syndrome, secondary to deletions affecting both genes, has been described. These patients are characterized by severe early onset of polycystic kidney disease.

INVESTIGATIONS

Ultrasonography, CT, and arteriography are the mainstay for the diagnosis and are helpful in distinguishing angiomyolipomas from renal cysts or tumors.

HISTOLOGY

Renal angiomyolipomas are hamartomas formed by atypical blood vessels, smooth muscle-like cells, and adipose tissue. Cysts originate from any nephron segment. The epithelium lining of the cysts exhibits marked cellular hypertrophy and hyperplasia.

PROGNOSIS

Affected patients frequently have early onset of severe hypertension and chronic renal failure that progress to end-stage renal failure in the second or third decade of life. Patients who develop end-stage renal failure are candidates for renal transplantation. Immunosuppressive therapy does not worsen the course of TSC.

MANAGEMENT

Renal angiomyolipomas are usually asymptomatic and require no treatment. Aggressive control of blood pressure may slow renal disease progression. Patients with TSC are at increased risk for developing renal tumors and need to be followed on a yearly basis with a CT or renal ultrasound.

Table 11 NIH consensus panel for TSC diagnostic criteria

Major features
- Facial angiofibromas
- Periungual fibroma
- Ash-leaf spots (>3)
- Shagreen patch
- Retinal hamartomas
- Subependymal nodule
- Giant cell astrocytoma
- Cardiac rhabdomyoma
- Cortical tuber†
- Lymphangiomyomatosis‡
- Renal angiomyolipomas‡

Minor features
- Gingival fibromas
- Nonrenal hamartomas
- Multiple renal cysts§
- Bone cysts‼
- Hamartomatous rectal polyps§
- Cerebral white matter migration lines†‼

Minor features (continued)
- Dental enamel pits
- Confetti macules

Definite diagnosis: either 2 major feature or 1 major feature with 2 minor features.
Probable diagnosis: 1 major feature and 1 minor feature
Possible diagnosis: either 1 major or 2 more minor features

† Cortical dysplasia and cerebral white matter migration occurring together should be counted as 1 rather than 2 features of TSC.
‡ Simultaneous occurrence of lymphangiomyomatosis and renal angiomyolipomas requires other features of TSC to be present before a definitive diagnosis is assigned.
§ Histologic confirmation is recommended
‼ Radiologic confirmation is sufficient

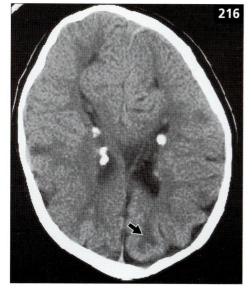

216 Head CT without contrast showing calcified subependymal nodules and a cortical/subcortical tuber in the right frontal lobe (arrow).

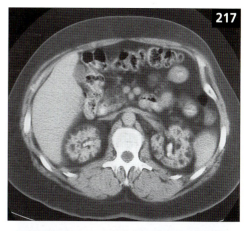

217 Multiple angiomyolipomas.

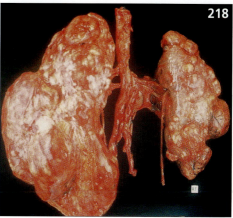

218 Markedly distended kidneys due to multiple angiomyolipomas.

Chapter Eight

Tumors of the renal parenchyma and urothelium

- **Introduction**

- **Tumors of the renal parenchyma**

- **Renal urothelial tumors**

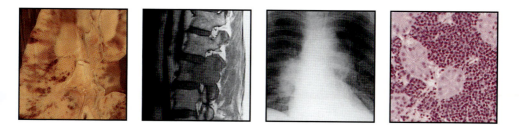

Introduction

Most renal tumors are malignant in childhood and adult life. Benign simple cysts of the renal parenchyma are seen with increasing frequency over the age of 50 years (**219**). Macroscopic hematuria, pain, and weight loss are the three commonest symptoms experienced in cases of renal malignancy. Imaging techniques for the primary tumor include ultrasound, CT, MRI, angiography, and retrograde ureteroscopy. Metastatic spread to lung, bone, and lymph nodes is commonplace. Direct spread into surrounding tissues, or invasion into the renal vein (and even into the right atrium) is a predilection shown by renal cell carcinoma.

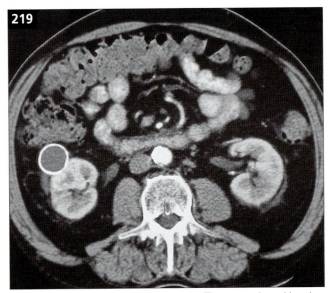

219 CT scan of the kidneys with contrast. The antero-lateral border of the right kidney is distorted by the presence of a large single simple renal cyst with a calcified wall.

Tumors of the renal parenchyma

CHILDHOOD TUMORS
Wilm's tumor (nephroblastoma)
The peak age incidence for this tumor is 2 years, but onset from age 1–10 years is not unusual (**220**). The overall incidence world-wide is about 5 per million children under the age of 15 years. Presenting features include a visible/palpable mass, hematuria, and weight loss (or failure to grow). Surgery to remove the tumor is the definitive treatment. The tumor is usually large by the time it presents and has a pale firm cut surface (with islands of darker hemorrhage and necrosis). There is an immature spindle-cell stroma which surrounds primitive tubular and glomerular structures on micro-scopy (**221**, **222**). Radiotherapy and chemo-therapy are extremely important adjunctive therapies. The cure rate in specialized centers is currently 80–90%.

Mesoblastic nephroma
These tumors typically occur within the first 6 months of life and are very rare after 12 months. Their cut surface is whorled like a uterine fibroid. Surgery alone usually lead to a cure.

Multicystic nephroma
This presents as a very well-defined multicystic mass involving one but not both kidneys in early childhood. Surgery alone will effect a cure.

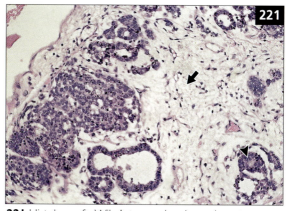

221 Histology of a Wilm's tumor showing an immature spindle-cell stroma (arrow) which surrounds primitive tubular and glomerular structures (arrow head) on microscopy (H+E x200).

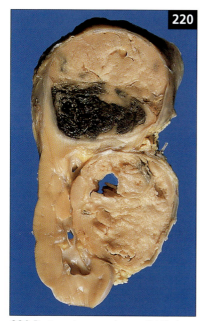

220 Postmortem specimen of Wilm's tumor in a child. The tumor is usually large by the time it presents and has a pale firm cut surface (with islands of darker hemorrhage and necrosis).

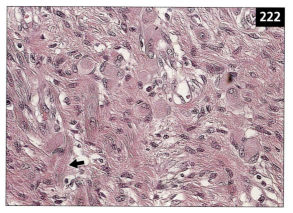

222 Histology of a Wilm's tumor showing muscle differentiation (with cross striations visible at the arrow) (H+E x400).

Tumors of the renal parenchyma (*continued*)

ADULT TUMORS
Renal cell carcinoma (hypernephroma)
This is the commonest renal tumor with an annual incidence of 5/100,000 population. The cut surface of a renal cell tumor is pale yellow with black areas of hemorrhage (**223, 224**). It is commonest between the fifth and seventh decades of life, but can occur earlier, especially in the clinical context of von Hippel–Lindau disease (see Chapter 7). Presentation with renal cell carcinoma is most often with frank hematuria, flank pain, and weight loss. Metabolic consequences of the tumor such as hypercalcemia, fever, or polycythemia are well-recognized but rare.

Ultrasound, CT and MRI scanning, and arteriography help to delineate the size and disposition of the primary tumor (**225**), and local spread including invasion of the inferior vena cava by extension along the renal vein (**226**). A chest film and CT (**227, 228**) are important as one-third of tumors have already metastasized by diagnosis; distant metastases are common, and often involve the skin and bones (**229, 230**). Bleeding, pathologic fracture, and pain are features of distant metastatic disease (**231, 232**).

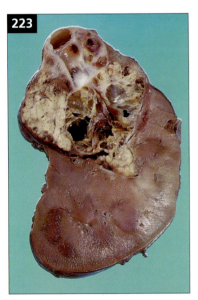

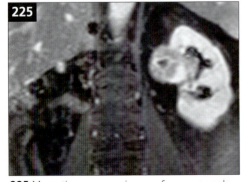

223 Postmortem specimens of a 'hypernephroma' (clear cell renal carcinoma) arising from the upper renal pole.

224 'Hypernephroma' arising from the lower renal pole.

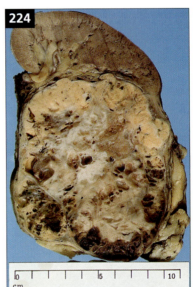

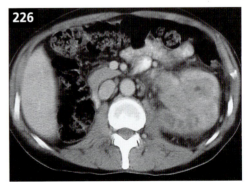

225 Magnetic resonance image of an upper-pole renal cell carcinoma.

226 CT scan of a clear cell renal carcinoma (occupying most of the enlarged single kidney) showing invasion of the inferior vena cava.

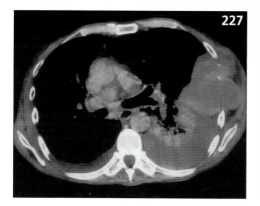

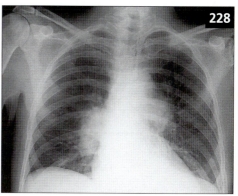

227 CT scan of thorax showing a large soft tissue mass eroding through ribs and emerging onto the chest wall.

228 Plain CXR showing hugely enlarged hilar lymph nodes.

229 AP plain radiograph of lumbar spine showing a missing vertebral pedicle (arrow).

230 MRI of lumbar spine showing vertebral body destruction by metastatic renal cell carcinoma (arrow).

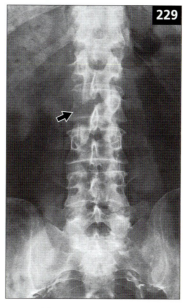

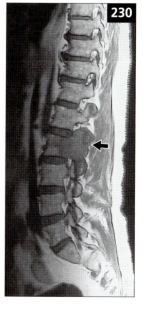

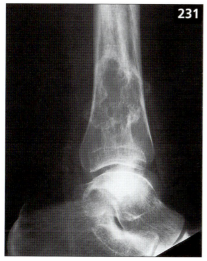

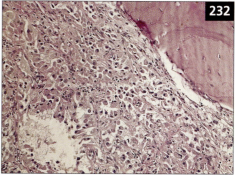

231, 232 Pathological tumor deposit expanding the cortex of the lower tibia (**231**). Postmortem histology (**232**) from the bone marrow showing diffuse infiltration by monomorphic malignant cells (renal cell carcinoma) (H+E ×100).

Tumors of the renal parenchyma (*continued*)

A single tumor can show marked variation in histology (**233**) from papillary growth pattern to anaplastic sarcoma-like stroma.

The standard surgical intervention is radical nephrectomy (removing kidney, adrenal, upper ureter and perirenal fascial/fat planes). Adjunctive chemotherapy and radiotherapy (the latter especially for distant metastases to control pain) are palliative.

Progesterone therapy is only modestly effective in slowing tumor growth in some patients. Interferon therapy, and removing the primary tumor, may be more effective. The tumor can be very slow growing.

Renal cell adenoma
These are small tumors that resemble renal cell carcinomas, but have a consistent histologic pattern, e.g. papillary. These are often incidentally located, or removed with a nephrectomy. They have very little malignant potential.

Renal oncocytoma
Oncocytes are cells with an eosinophilic granular cytoplasm. These tumors can grow to a large size but rarely metastasize (**234, 235**).

Angiomyolipomata
These tumors are highly vascular but also contain smooth muscle and fat components as well as those from blood vessels (**236, 237**). There is a strong association with tuberous sclerosis (and see Chapter 7). These tumors can grow large enough to be palpable and present as a mass. Hemorrhage into these vascular tumors, with pain and anemia, is common as these tumors exceed 5 cm (2 in) in diameter. Nephron-sparing surgery can be undertaken successfully.

Renal lymphoma/leukemia
A primary renal lymphoma (usually B-cell) is exceptionally rare. Lymphomatous or leukematous involvement of the kidneys is rare but not so uncommon in chronic lymphatic leukemia (up to 20% of CLL cases at postmortem can have renal deposits) (**238–241**). Post-transplantation lymphoproliferative disease (see Chapter 12) can affect the allograft.

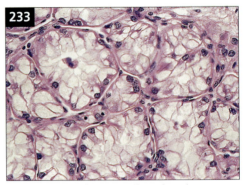

233 Histology of a 'clear cell' renal carcinoma showing tumor cells with abundant clear cytoplasm (containing fat) (H+E ×400).

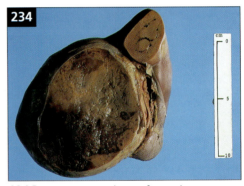

234 Postmortem specimen of a renal oncocytoma. The huge tumor has virtually replaced the normal renal tissue.

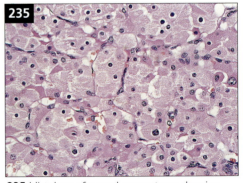

235 Histology of a renal oncocytoma showing eosinophilic granular cytoplasm (H+E ×400).

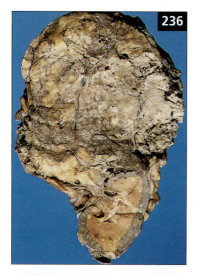

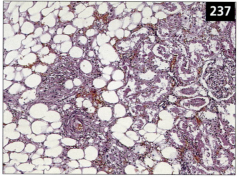

237 Histology of a renal angiomyolipoma. Abundant fat (clear areas) can be seen (H+E ×200).

236 Postmortem specimen of a large angiomyolipoma (a tumor composed of blood vessel, muscle, and fat) seen particularly in tuberous sclerosis.

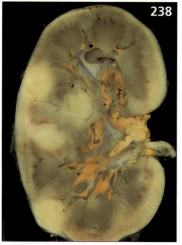

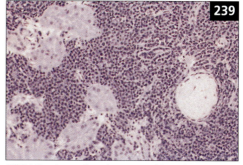

239 Histology of a primary renal lymphoma (consisting of an infiltrate of mononuclear lymphoid series cells) (H+E ×400).

238 Postmortem specimen of a kidney infiltrated (white areas) by metastatic lymphoma.

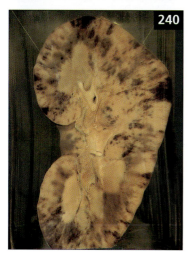

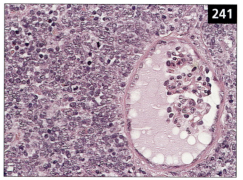

241 Histology of kidney infiltrated by acute lymphoblastic leukemia (H+E ×400).

240 Postmortem specimen of a kidney diffusely infiltrated (hemorrhagic areas) by acute lymphoblastic leukemia.

Renal urothelial tumors

The urothelium is a transitional epithelium from the renal papillae down to the urethra. Chemical carcinogens (rubber and aniline dye workers; cyclophosphamide therapy; phenacetin; thorotrast) and chronic inflammation (e.g. bilharzia, Chapter 6) are the main predisposing factors. About 10% of urothelial tumors occur in the upper tracts (renal pelvis and ureters) (242–245). They can present with hematuria, or obstruction. Malignant cells are seen on cytologic examination of the urine. Ureteroscopy and biopsy are also used in the diagnosis of upper tract tumors.

Removal of as much of the urothelium as possible is required, as the scope for future malignancy is very great.

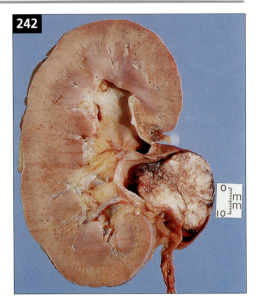

242 Postmortem appearance of a large tumor arising from the transitional epithelium in the renal pelvis.

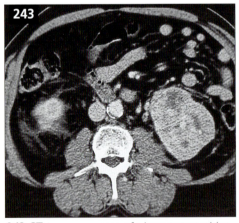

243 CT scan appearance of a large tumor arising from the transitional epithelium in the renal pelvis.

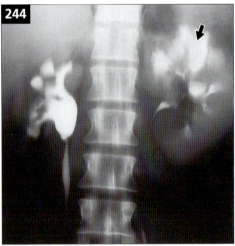

244 IVU appearance of a pelvic transitional cell carcinoma in the left kidney. The right kidney's pelvis and proximal ureter are full of radio-opaque contrast material. On the left there is virtually no contrast in the pelvis (a little is seen in the proximal ureter) which is radiolucent. The upper pole has significant patchy parenchymal contrast retention (arrow) compared to the lower pole and the contralateral kidney, due to partial obstruction at the level of the renal pelvis.

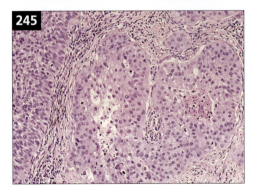

245 Histology of a transitional cell renal tumor showing malignant urothelial cells (H+E x400).

Chapter Nine

Renal disease in pregnancy

- **Normal pregnancy**

- **Renal diseases associated with pregnancy**

- **Pre-eclampsia**

- **Pregnancy in renal disease**

- **Pregnancy in dialysis patients**

- **Pregnancy in renal transplant patients**

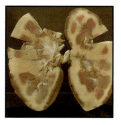
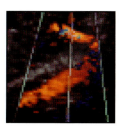
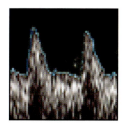
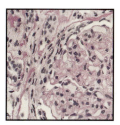

Normal pregnancy

During a normal gestation the kidneys enlarge in size and the renal calyces, pelves, and ureters become dilated due to hormonal effects on smooth muscle and possibly compression by the uterus. The right ureter is usually more dilated than the left. GFR increases by about 50% in the first trimester and remains at this level until delivery, thus lowering serum urea and creatinine levels. Blood pressure decreases early in pregnancy so that the diastolic pressure falls by 10–15 mmHg (1.3–2 kPa) by the 20th week, before slowly rising during the second half of pregnancy to approach prepregnancy levels at term.

Renal diseases associated with pregnancy

Urinary tract infections are common in pregnancy. Women with asymptomatic bacteriuria are likely to develop symptomatic infections in pregnancy, and should be treated with a course of antibiotics. Acute pyelonephritis in pregnancy is a serious complication and should be managed aggressively, in hospital with a prolonged course of antibiotics.

Acute renal failure in pregnancy may occur due to septic shock complicating acute pyelonephritis or septic abortions, or following hemorrhage or severe pre-eclampsia. Rare cases of acute renal failure are due to amniotic fluid embolism, acute fatty liver of pregnancy, and postpartum hemolytic uremic syndrome. Obstetric complications are the most common causes of acute cortical necrosis, the most severe outcome of acute renal failure (**246**). Acute cortical necrosis is most common in the last trimester, most frequently after placental abruption and less commonly following prolonged intra-uterine death or with pre-eclampsia. It may involve the entire renal cortex with irreversible renal failure, or be patchy with some return of renal function.

Pre-eclampsia

DEFINITION
Pre-eclampsia is characterized by hypertension, proteinuria, edema and, sometimes, liver function and coagulation abnormalities. It usually occurs in the last trimester. Eclampsia is characterized by grand-mal seizures.

EPIDEMIOLOGY AND ETIOLOGY
Pre-eclampsia occurs in 5–10% of all pregnancies and is most common in women having their first pregnancy. Other risk factors include a previous pregnancy complicated by pre-eclampsia, maternal age >35 years, twin pregnancy, diabetes mellitus, and pre-existing renal impairment (serum creatinine >1.5 mg/dl [133 μmol/l]).

PATHOGENESIS
Uteroplacental ischemia due to abnormal trophoblast implantation is thought to be the primary abnormality. There is increased peripheral resistance due to vasoconstriction, in part due to reduced prostacyclin production.

CLINICAL HISTORY
Pre-eclampsia may develop slowly or present abruptly. It occurs most commonly in the last trimester but may occasionally occur as early as 20 weeks. Edema with nephrotic range proteinuria is common. Headaches, epigastric pain, and vomiting often precede eclamptic fits.

INVESTIGATIONS
Hyperuricemia, deranged liver function tests, thombocytopenia, and coagulation disturbances may be seen. Renal biopsy is occasionally indicated in women with nephrotic syndrome when it is impossible clinically to distinguish between pre-eclampsia and a primary renal disease. Uterine artery Doppler ultrasound is useful in predicting women at risk of developing pre-eclampsia (**247**).

HISTOLOGY (248)
The glomeruli are enlarged due to swelling of glomerular endothelial cells ('glomerular endotheliosis'). The epithelial cells are normal. Deposits of IgM and fibrin are found. These changes reverse rapidly after delivery.

246 Acute cortical necrosis. Hemorrhagic zone can be seen affecting the outer 3–5 mm (0.1–0.2 in) of the renal cortex.

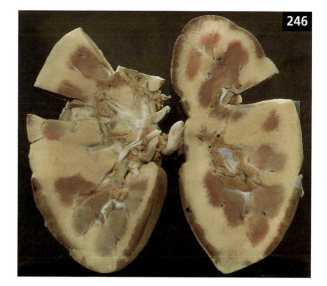

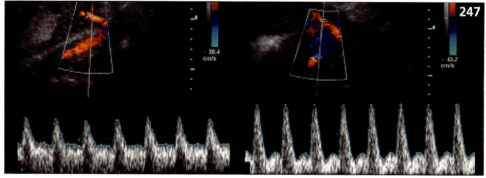

247 Normal (left) and abnormal (right) uterine artery Doppler ultrasound waveforms.

PROGNOSIS

Pre-eclampsia rapidly resolves after delivery. It is still the major cause of maternal death in the UK, with cerebral hemorrhage, pulmonary edema, and hepatic necrosis major causes of death. Pre-eclampsia is associated with fetal growth retardation, prematurity, miscarriage, and neurodevelopmental abnormalities.

MANAGEMENT

Definitive treatment is by delivery. Magnesium sulfate is the treatment of choice for seizures. Methyldopa, labetalol and hydralazine are effective antihypertensive agents in this condition. Aspirin and possibly antioxidant vitamins C and E may be useful prophylactic agents.

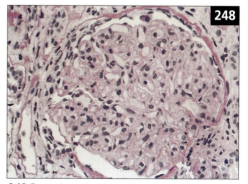

248 Pre-eclampsia. Light microscopy showing occlusion of glomerular capillary lumen by swelling of glomerular endothelial cells (H+E ×400).

Pregnancy in renal disease

Pre-existing renal disease can affect the outcome of pregnancy and pregnancy can alter the course of renal disease. Hypertension, heavy protein-uria, and impaired renal function all predispose to pre-eclampsia and prematurity. Pregnancy can accelerate the progression of renal failure, especially in patients with a creatinine >2.0 mg/dl (177 µmol/l) prior to pregnancy. In patients with chronic glomerulonephritis, pregnancy does not seem to worsen renal outcome if pre-existing renal function is good. The normal physiologic changes of pregnancy will increase the degree of proteinuria. Systemic lupus erythematosus commonly affects women of childbearing age, and pregnancy can cause complex clinical problems. Pregnancy may be associated with disease flares especially in the puerperium. Women with active SLE are advised not to conceive until the disease is under control. Mycophenolate mofetil is showing increasing promise in the treatment of lupus nephritis, but women are currently advised not to conceive whilst taking this drug because of concerns about teratogenicity. Anti-phospho-lipid antibodies are associated with fetal loss in all three trimesters and with pre-eclampsia.

Prepregnancy counseling is essential to explain the risks of pregnancy in patients with renal disease.

Pregnancy in dialysis patients

Pregnancy is rare in dialysis patients because of reduced libido and impaired fertility. The risks need to be carefully explained to the parents: maternal hypertension, pre-eclampsia, pre-maturity, and intra-uterine growth retardation. If the parents decide to proceed with the pregnancy very careful monitoring of mother and fetus is required, with aggressive dialysis essential (*Table 12*). Dialysis aims to keep blood urea below 15 mmol/l (90 mg/dl), control hypertension, and minimize hypotension during dialysis which could reduce placental blood flow. Therefore daily hemodialysis is optimal.

Pregnancy in renal transplant patients

The outcome is excellent for pregnancy in women with stable and good renal transplant function. Women with chronic renal failure should thus be advised to defer pregnancy until they have been successfully transplanted.

Women with impaired graft function are at increased risk of pre-eclampsia and worsening renal function with pregnancy. The guidelines for preconception counseling for renal transplant patients are listed in *Table 13*.

Table 12 Guidelines to optimize pregnancy outcome in the dialysis patient

- Prophylactic dialysis: urea <15 mmol/l (90 mg/dl) to avoid polyhydramnios
- HD: 5–7 sessions/week, bicarbonate, minimal heparin, slow ultrafiltration
- PD: decrease volumes and increase frequency
- Adequate supply of calories and protein
  Protein intake 1 g/kg/day + 20 g/day for fetal growth
  Water soluble vitamins/zinc
- Tight BP control with methyldopa and beta blockers
- Correction of anemia
  Hb 10–11; erythropoietin, iron, and folic acid
- Prevention of metabolic acidosis
- Prevention of hypocalcemia with calcium carbonate
- Treatment of premature labor
  Use beta agonist; avoid NSAIDs
- Regular fetal monitoring

Table 13 Guidelines for preconception counseling in renal transplant recipients

- Wait at least 1 year post-transplant
- Stable good renal function
- No recent rejection
- Minimal proteinuria
- Absence of pelvicalyceal distension
- Easily managed hypertension
- Drug therapy reduced to maintenance levels
- Avoid mycophenolate mofetil, sirolimus

Chapter Ten

Acute renal failure

- **Introduction**

- **Epidemiology**

- **Classification**

- **Clinical assessment**

- **Management and outcome**

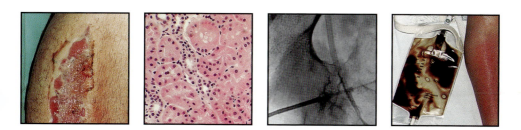

Introduction

Acute renal failure (ARF) is a medical emergency which taxes both the patient and the physician alike. ARF is likely to be encountered in the community and in hospital wards and intensive care units, with input from generalists, internal medicine specialists, cardiologists, diabetologists, infectious disease specialists, gerentologists, general, orthopedic, vascular and cardiothoracic surgeons, and obstetricians – and of course, nephrologists.

ARF is not one disease, but a stereotyped renal response to myriad different renal insults, with different pathophysiologic mechanisms. ARF can arise alone, or in the context of two, three, or four organ failures (**249, 250**). Many of the renal insults that end up causing ARF are the result of modern medicine and surgery – there is some opportunity for prediction and prevention (not always grasped). Equally, prompt detection and diagnosis of ARF can arrest an otherwise inevitable cycle of events that leads to protracted renal shut-down and the need for dialysis, with the attendant increase in mortality.

DEFINITION OF ARF

Arbitrarily ARF is defined as a rapid and substantial decline in excretory renal function (i.e. sudden fall in GFR) leading to accumulation of nitrogenous waste products and electrolytes. There is no broadly-accepted definition of the degree of renal impairment (i.e. rise in urea or creatinine), nor its rapidity of onset.

Epidemiology

The lack of a precise consensus definition of ARF makes for difficulties comparing epidemiologic ARF series. If one includes any case of minor reversible alteration in renal function – seen by any physician, not necessarily dialysed – the incidence is probably 200–300 cases per million population per year; the figure is about 50 cases for those requiring dialysis. In major tertiary hospitals 5% of inpatients may develop ARF (reflecting the types of surgery and medicine practiced, e.g. coronary interventions, vascular surgery).

The incidence of ARF rises very steeply with age for three reasons. First, older patients have a greater number of comorbidities, whose treatment may well be the cause of ARF: second, because natural defence mechanisms, such as cardiovascular reflexes, autoregulation, and anti-bacterial and anti-oxidant systems are less effective: and third, because from the age of 40 years GFR declines by about 9 ml/min/decade – a subject aged 80 years will have about 50% of the renal function of someone 50 years or so younger.

In the hospital setting acute tubular necrosis is by far the commonest cause of ARF (roughly evenly divided between sepsis and ischemia) but, in the community, prostatic obstruction and drugs are the main causes of ARF. The increasing use of nonsteroidal anti-inflammatories, and ACE inhibitors and angiotensin receptor blockers, often in an aging population, is a major factor in community-acquired ARF.

In developing countries, obstetric, infective and toxic causes of ARF predominate.

249, 250 Patients in an intensive care setting with multiple organ failure after trauma or surgery. Acute renal failure is common. **249** shows a wide defect in the anterior abdominal wall after surgery for necrotising fasciitis. **250** shows a road traffic accident victim.

Classification

Traditionally and usefully ARF is classified into prerenal (hemodynamic), renal, and postrenal causes. This classification provides a conceptual framework for the understanding of ARF and its management. *Table 14* lists the major causations arranged logically and mechanistically.

Table 14 Classification of causes of acute renal failure		
ARF classification	*Mechanism*	*Example*
Prerenal	Reduced effective circulating blood volume	GI bleed Pancreatitis Hypotension Sepsis
Renal	Renal arterial occlusion	Thrombosis Embolism Ligation
	Small vessel disease	Vasculitis HUS/TTP Embolic Hypertension Scleroderma
	Interstitial disease	Drugs Autoimmune Infection Malignancy
	Glomerulonephritis	Lupus Rapidly progressive glomerulonephritis
	Ischemic ATN	Many Maintained prerenal
	Toxic ATN: endogenous	Rhabdomyolysis Bilirubin Hemoglobin Light chains
	Toxic ATN: exogenous	Drugs Contrast media
	Intratubular blockage	Casts Crystals
	Renal vein occlusion	Nephrotic syndrome
Postrenal	Obstruction	Prostate Ureter

Classification (*continued*)

PRERENAL ARF
Pathophysiology of prerenal ARF
The fundamental change is a marked reduction in glomerular perfusion. Decreased effective circulating blood volume is the major reason for this. A number of factors can cause this change – the most common is hypovolemia which itself has many causations. Congestive cardiac failure, cirrhosis, sepsis, and severe nephrotic syndrome can act similarly.

Normally baroreceptors and baroreflexes act to maintain perfusion pressures. As these are activated, the renin–angiotensin and sympathetic nervous systems are activated, and ADH released. Systemic vasoconstriction occurs but renal arterial resistance rises to a lesser extent. Renal blood flow is highly regulated to achieve constancy by autoregulation (myogenic reflex) across the mean arterial pressure range of 60–160 mmHg (8–21.3 kPa) in health. As well as this autoregulation the kidney can autoregulate GFR and blood flow simultaneously; this is achieved by having independent mechanisms to control the tone of the afferent and efferent arterioles. Angiotensin, prostaglandins, nitric oxide, and other vascular mediators have crucial roles in these tasks.

All of the above devices and mechanisms have limits beyond which renal injury cannot be prevented. Once efferent arterioles start to constrict (e.g. with very profound sympathetic nervous system activation), renal blood flow and GFR fall and renal failure ensues.

Causes of prerenal ARF
These include hypovolemia (blood or urine or fluid loss) and contributions from inadequate salt and water intake. Left ventricular failure (LVF) is a cause of prerenal ARF, as is overzealous use of diuretics or ACE inhibitors to treat LVF. Cirrhosis of the liver is associated with systemic and intrarenal hemodynamic derangements – in part because of abnormal prostanoid generation and handling. Hypoalbuminemia may also play a role, as it more clearly does in the ARF seen rarely in severe nephrotic syndrome. ACE inhibitors and angiotensin receptor blockers can induce ARF in patients whose GFR is maintained only by angiotensin-II-mediated efferent arteriolar vasoconstriction. This is seen especially with a hemodynamically significant renal artery stenosis (stenosis >80%, see Chapter 5), but can also be seen in cirrhosis and heart failure. The abrupt change in GFR is seen only with a severe stenosis affecting a single functional kidney, or with bilateral stenoses. GFR can be rapidly restored to normal by withdrawl of the drug, though rarely thrombosis of the renal artery can occur in a low-blood flow/acute illness setting.

Nonsteroidal anti-inflammatories (NSAIDs) profoundly inhibit prostaglandin synthesis. In a variable but small number of people renal blood flow is exquisitely dependent on endothelially-derived renal prostanoids. In a setting of low effective circulating volume (e.g. sepsis, diarrhea), or with other nephrotoxic drugs, NSAIDS can cause ARF.

Cyclosporine (cyclosporin) usually causes intense afferent arteriolar vasoconstriction and leads to a fall in GFR. The vasoconstriction seems to be multifactorial and related to reduced NO production, to greater endothelin and thromboxane production, and activation of the renin–angiotensin and sympathetic nervous systems. Early withdrawal of cyclosporine (cyclosporin) leads to rapid GFR recovery; later, interstitial fibrosis leads to long-term loss of GFR.

RENAL/PARENCHYMAL ARF
Acute tubular necrosis (ATN)
Pathophysiology of ATN
ATN describes the injury to the renal parenchyma that occurs following prolonged renal ischemia or exposure to nephrotoxins. The term ATN is of course histologic but typically inferential – ironically it is this type of patient who is least likely to undergo renal biopsy as potentially ATN is recoverable; the acute necrosis of renal tubular epithelial cells is followed by tubular regeneration.

The proximal tubule and the medullary thick ascending loop of Henle are the most susceptible areas to injury. In part this is because the renal medulla is intensely metabolically active (the S3 tubular segments especially so), receives only 20% of renal blood flow (normal renal blood flow is 1200 ml/min), and is incipiently hypoxic even in health (oxygen tension is typically 3–4 kPa [22.5– 30 mmHg]). Decreased oxygenation or increased metabolic demand can lead to hypoxic damage.

Necrosis and apoptosis are seen in the tubules as lethal cell changes (**251–256**). Less severe damage causes cell swelling, vacuolation, disruption of the tubular cell cytoskeleton, dissolution of the integrin-dependent cell matrix adhesion, loss of cell surface brush border, and cell desquamation into the tubular lumen. Thus cellular debris is shed into the proximal renal

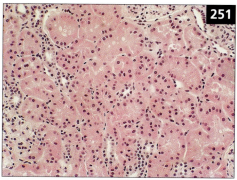

251 Histology of normal renal tubules. Note 'back-to-back' renal tubules with plump epithelial cells (H+E ×150).

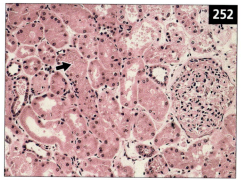

252 Acute tubular necrosis. Desquamated epithelial cells causes tubular blockage (arrow) (H+E ×200).

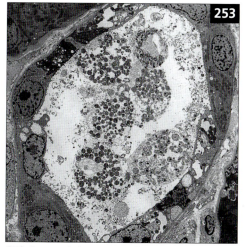

253 Acute tubular necrosis. Electron micrograph of a proximal tubule showing blockage with cellular debris.

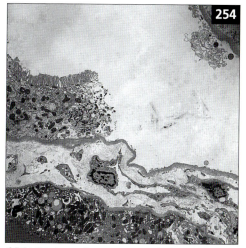

254 Histology of severe acute tubular necrosis. Electron micrograph of a tubule showing rupture/destruction of the delicate brush border.

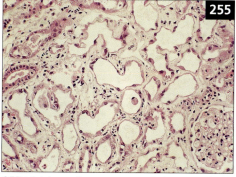

255 Histology of severe acute tubular necrosis, with widespread renal tubular epithelial cell attenuation (H+E ×250).

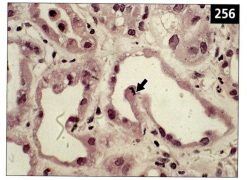

256 Histology of milder/recovering ATN. Tubular epithelial cell regeneration is seen (mitotic figures) (arrow) (H+E ×400).

Classification (*continued*)

tubules and this debris can block the distal tubules once it has combined with the viscid Tamm–Horsfall protein secreted there. Light chains in myeloma (**59**) or myoglobin in rhabdomyolysis form 'hard' casts which plug distal tubules, and may excite an inflammatory reaction in surrounding parenchyma.

Recovery of ATN requires tubular regeneration and luminal patency. Understanding how to manipulate these processes may one day reap rich clinical dividends.

ACUTE CORTICAL NECROSIS

Unlike ATN, cortical necrosis (**246**) is virtually impossible to recover from. There is microvascular and glomerular thrombosis and cortical infarction. Medullary blood supply can be maintained (but to no useful purpose). Obstetric emergencies (abruptio placentae), endotoxinemia and DIC are typical causes of this very rare outcome to acute renal injury. Why some patients develop ATN and not cortical necrosis or *vice versa* is not clear. Children seem more prone to cortical necrosis than do adults.

Though the classical appearance of tram-line renal cortical calcification is well-known (and can also be seen on CT scanning) (**257–259**), in practice this is unusual, and renal biopsy is a more reliable way to determine its presence.

RAPIDLY PROGRESSIVE GLOMERULONEPHRITIS (RPGN)

Particularly out of hospital this can be an important cause of ARF and must be diagnosed in time for treatment to be effective. Red cell casts in the urine are pathognomonic, but not totally specific (**8**). Typically RPGN is due to renal or systemic vasculitis; often auto-antibodies or signs of inflammation are present. The urine tests strongly positive for blood and protein and the urinary sediment contains red cell casts. Renal biopsy is the best way to achieve a diagnosis. Treatment is typically with prednisolone, cyclophosphamide, and plasma exchange in some cases (Chapter 3).

ENDOGENOUS NEPHROTOXINS

Myoglobinuria and acute myoglobinuric renal failure were first described in the context of air-raid bomb damage victims. Rhabdomyolysis is a fairly common cause of ATN, seen in 5–10% of hospitalized cases.

Myoglobin is a freely-filtered 17 kDa heme-protein which is normally endocytically re-absorbed in the proximal tubule but in gross excess these defences are overwhelmed and a great load of myoglobin is received in the distal tubule, where it precipitates to block the tubule (particularly in acid urine [**260**]) and causes oxidative damage (the heme scavenges NO). Rhabdomyolysis patients often have severe volume depletion (as their muscles are grossly edematous). This is an example of several mechanisms combining to produce renal injury.

Trauma remains an important etiology, but muscle damage from pressure (e.g. alcoholic stupor, or coma) is more common. Status epilepticus or neuroleptic malignant syndrome can also induce severe muscle damage. Marathon running in an undertrained dehydrated individual is another risk for this type of problem. Drug reactions (e.g. statins, fibrates) are seen rarely; rhabdomyolysis is seen in <0.1% patients on statins. Intense myositis (viral, immune) or inherited muscle enzyme defects such as McCardle's syndrome (myophosphorylase deficiency) or carnitine palmityl transferase deficiency complete the picture.

Muscles are usually swollen, painful, and tender – indeed fasciotomies may be needed quickly if a limb is to retain viability (**261**). Urine is chocolate-brown in color (**262**). The urine dipstick shows intense heme reaction, but microscopy does not show any red blood cells. The urine myoglobin should be measured, as should plasma creatine phosphokinase (invariably elevated >5000 U/ml). Creatinine, uric acid, phosphate, potassium, and acid moieties are all released from dead muscle. Hypocalcemia in the acute phase is common; hypercalcemia in the recovery phase is rarer.

Treatment is by means of adequate hydration by intravenous infusion of saline and dilute bicarbonate. Dialysis or filtration may be needed to prevent lethal hyperkalemia, or to remove a causative factor, e.g. theophylline leading to status epilepticus and muscle damage. Recovery is usual within 3 weeks; there are no long-term renal sequelae.

Hemoglobinuric-ATN is seen in the context of massive intravascular hemolysis, e.g. glucose-6-phosphate deficiency, paroxysmal nocturnal hemoglobinuria, blood transfusion reaction, malaria, drugs, venoms, and prosthetic heart valves. Hemoglobin being much larger than myoglobin is much less well-filtered, and is less tubularly toxic.

The plasma is typically pink in hemoglobinuria; the urine can often be a normal color (though it is black when severe). Hydration and

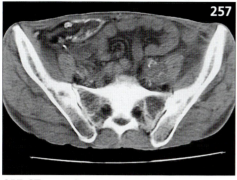

257 CT scan of a renal transplant showing diffuse calcification of a much-thinned renal cortex. The graft had been 'lost' many years before following DIC secondary to severe bacterial sepsis.

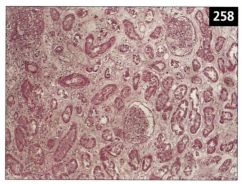

258 Histology of acute cortical necrosis showing pallor/infarction of tubules and glomeruli (H+E ×10).

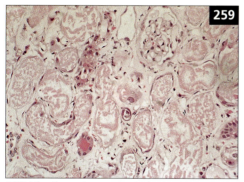

259 Histology of acute cortical necrosis showing survival of some endothelial cells (H+E ×250).

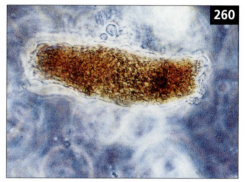

260 Myoglobin cast (chocolate-brown color) in urine (H+E ×300).

261 Muscle fasciotomy to prevent acute compartment syndrome in a case of acute rhabdomyolysis (following a prolonged stupor after alcohol excess).

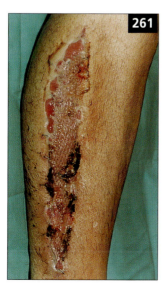

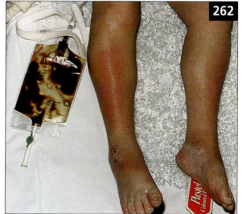

262 Chocolate-brown colored, thick urine in the catheter bag. Leg redness and edema can also be seen in this elderly female who fell at home and lay helpless for 48 hours on the floor.

Classification (*continued*)

urine alkalinization are recommended; obviously removing the cause of hemolysis is paramount.

Bilirubin causes ATN only when there is additional renal injury, e.g. sepsis – so ascending cholangitis would be a prime example. Relief of biliary obstruction, hydration, and vigorous treatment of sepsis are indicated (**263, 264**).

Some light chains are directly nephrotoxic; acute renal failure is a rare but important presentation of acute myeloma. Cast nephropathy can occur which evinces a brisk inflammatory reaction in the renal interstitium. Myeloma casts tend to be dense, fractured, and associated with a giant cell reaction (**59**).

Crystals can be seen in acute elevation of uric acid levels, e.g. after chemotherapy in tumor-lysis syndrome. Urine alkalinization and allo-purinol are needed urgently. Hypercalcemia can also cause intratubular crystal deposition.

EXOGENOUS NEPHROTOXINS

Ethylene glycol (antifreeze) is readily metabol-ized by alcohol dehydrogenase to glycolic acid, which is a tubular toxin, glyoaxalic, and oxalic acids. Oxaluria ensues with a metabolic acidosis. Oxalate crystals may precipitate intratubularly.

Alcohol, bicarbonate, and fomeprizole are treat-ments for this potentially lethal poisoning.

Contrast media are known for their nephro-toxicity despite the introduction over the last two decades of non-ionic media, which are substantially less toxic. However, many older subjects are undergoing studies involving the use of these agents. Age, diabetes, myeloma, use of metformin, and pre-existing renal failure are risk factors for renal damage.

The media are significantly hyperosmolar and impose an oxidative stress on tubules. Acute oliguria is unusual – more often there is gradual oliguria and renal impairment over 3–7 days postcontrast load. If there has been an aortogram or a cardiac catheter, atheroembolism from the vascular catheter in an atherosclerotic aorta, as well as contrast nephrotoxicity, can induce renal failure. Adequate hydration and N-acetyl cysteine are potential preventative measures.

Drugs are a very important cause of nephro-toxicity by a number of different mechanisms. Some drugs compromise the hemodynamic response to renal injury, other cause crystalluria, others cause acute renal parenchymal injury, e.g. acute interstitial nephritis (**108**). Reactions can be dose-dependent or idiosyncratic. *Table 15* lists the most important nephrotoxic drugs.

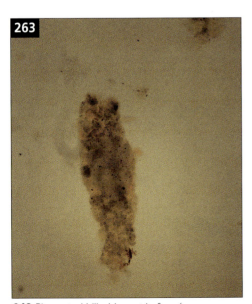

263 Pigmented bilirubin cast in free (green-colored) urine following acute severe drug-induced hemolytic anemia.

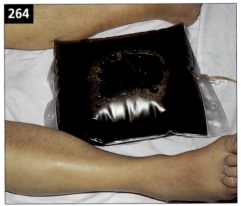

264 Deep-green jaundice, and deep-green peritoneal dialysate, from a patient in acute renal failure following acute, severe, drug-induced hemolytic anemia.

POSTRENAL ARF

By definition this is a urologic area. Pelvi-ureteric, ureteric, vesico-ureteric, bladder, prostate, and urethral obstruction can give rise to ARF. Prolonged obstruction leads to severe cortical thinning (265) and loss of renal function, so that relief of obstruction may not then be accompanied by worthwhile renal functional recovery.

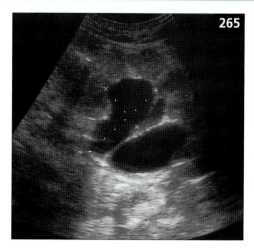

265

265 Ultrasound scan showing gross hydronephrosis and severe cortical thinning (**2–4**).

Table 15 Nephrotoxic drugs		
Classification/mechanism	**Example**	
Intrarenal vascular		
Thrombotic microangiopathy	Cyclosporine (cyclosporin), tacrolimus, mitomycin C, oral contraceptive pill	
Vasculitis	Amphetamines	
Toxic ATN		
Antimicrobials	Aminoglycosides	Amphotericin
	Vancomycin	Pentamidine
	Foscarnet	
Chemotherapy	Cisplatin	5-fluoruracil
	Ifosfamide	Cytarabine
	Mithramycin	
Miscellaneous	Lithium	
	Paracetamol (acetaminophen)	
Recreational drugs	Ecstasy	Amphetamines
Interstitial nephritis	Antibiotics	NSAIDs
Urinary tract obstruction		
Papillary necrosis	Analgesic, NSAIDs	
Crystals	Aciclovir (acyclovir)	Triamterine
	Methotrexate	Indinavir
	Sulfonamides	
Retroperitoneal fibrosis	Ergotamine	

Classification (*continued*)

Cases of obstruction can be much more subtle (**266–271**) (see also urinary tract obstruction in Chapter 6, p. 106). As an initial approach a nephrostomy can be inserted into a dilated pelvicalyceal system (the puncture can reveal pus or blood and not just urine). Urinary tract stenting may be needed. As well as relieving obstruction a nephrostomy can allow investigation of its causation (**272–274**). Dialysis sessions may still be needed for a while as accompanying ATN is common, especially if there have been nephrotoxic drugs in use, or sepsis. Teamwork between urologic and nephrologic specialists is essential.

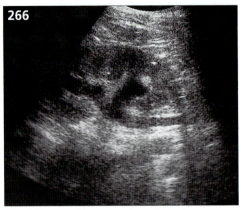

266 Ultrasound scan showing mild hydronephrosis and dilatation of the proximal ureter.

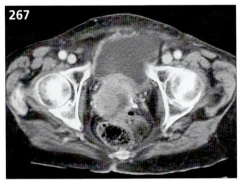

267 CT scan of the pelvis showing a large gynecological mass. This was responsible for acute renal failure in a 90-year-old female (same patient as **265, 266**).

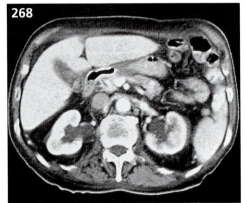

268 CT scan of the kidneys showing mild bilateral hydronephrosis.

269, 270 IVU from a female discovered to be in acute renal failure (and with anemia, back pain, and an ESR of >120 mm/first hour). Early phase (**269**) shows relatively normal nephrogram and pyelogram for the left kidney, but with medial indrawing of the left ureter. Right kidney is obstructed. Later phase (**270**) shows late retention of contrast in a dilated right renal pelvis, and marked proximal right ureteric medial indrawing. A case of retroperitoneal fibrosis.

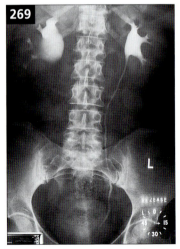

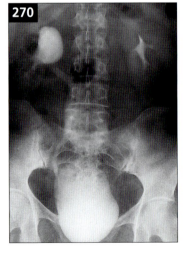

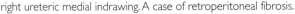

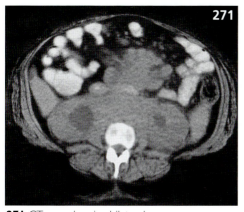

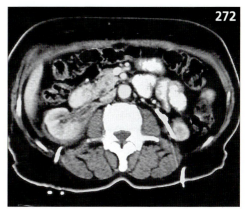

271 CT scan showing bilateral severe hydronephrosis, worse on the right. A large soft tissue mass is present between the kidneys arising from the retroperitoneum. Biopsy disclosed B-cell lymphoma.

272 Abdominal CT scan showing a small right kidney, a normal left kidney, and two percutaneous nephrostomies.

273 An antegrade contrast study (antegrade pyelography) where contrast is injected down the nephrostomy tube into the renal pelvis. The contrast in this case terminates abruptly at the lower ureter near the vesicoureteric junction. This is a typical site for tumors.

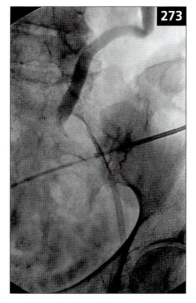

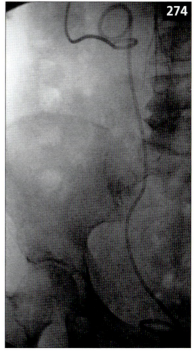

274 A nephrostomy can be seen entering the renal pelvis, and then a ureteric stent can be seen from renal pelvis down the ureter to the bladder.

Clinical assessment (*Table 16*)

As there are so many different causes of ARF, there needs to be a logical exercise in information and evidence gathering, assimilating diverse information, then answering some basic fundamental questions, the answers to which give insight into causation and appropriate intervention:
- Is this acute renal failure (i.e. was there normal or abnormal renal function before)?
- Is there evidence of reduction in circulating blood volume?
- Has there been a major vascular occlusion?
- Are there clearly identifiable nephrotoxins?
- Is there parenchymal disease other than ATN?
- Is there any evidence of renal tract obstruction?

The assessment of the patient must be thorough enough to answer all of these points. Thus, most of the following are often needed:
- Complete physical examination (volume, icterus, ascites, bruits).
- Careful scrutiny of old notes, drug and fluid charts, computer records.
- Urinalysis, urine volume, biochemistry.
- Blood tests (renal, liver, immunologic, hematologic).
- Renal tract imaging – plain film, ultrasound, CT scan, nuclear medicine.
- Renal angiography.
- Renal biopsy.

Table 16 Differentiating features of investigations into ARF

Assessment	Prerenal	ATN	Acute GN	Interstitial	Atheroembolic	Obstruction
Clinical	Hypovolemia	Ischemic toxin	Rare anuria	Drugs, rash eosinophils	Vasculopathy	Pain, anuria
Urea/creatinine ratio	High	Medium	Medium	Medium	Medium	High
Urinary sodium* (mmol/l [mEq/l])	<10	>50	<10	10–100	>50	<20
Urinalysis	Normal	Casts	+++ bld +++ prot	+bld +prot WBC eosinophils	Normal	Normal
Urine osmolality* (mmol/kg [mOsm/kg] H_2O)	>500	<350	300–500	300–500	<350	>500
Ultrasound size	Normal	Normal	Enlarged	Normal	Scars/small	Pelvis and calyces dilated

*Urine osmolality and electrolyte data are uninterpretable in the presence of loop diuretics

Management and outcome

PRERENAL ARF

To restore depleted intravascular volume the choice is between blood and isotonic solutions (saline or Ringer's). Colloid versus crystalloid has been a recently controversial question – there seem to be few real advantages to the more expensive colloids. Patients can often have salt and water overload (extracellular salt and water excess) while being intravascularly volume depleted. Salt and water diuresis must be matched by movement from the extracellular to the intravascular spaces, otherwise further volume depletion will occur. Loop diuretics, as either a bolus or an infusion, with, in refractory cases, salt-poor albumin, can be effective. Improving heart failure-induced ARF involves a twin strategy of increasing cardiac output and reducing cardiac afterload, e.g. inotropes and nitrates. Noradrenaline (norepinephrine) to 'tighten' the excessively vasodilated systemic circulation can be effective in 'sepsis' ARF (but needs careful monitoring of cardiac output and systemic vascular resistance). Dopamine has been in vogue (whether at high dose as an alpha agonist or at so-called 'low dose' as a renal vasodilator) for three decades. Sadly there never has been any evidence that using dopamine is helpful; there is quite a lot of evidence that it is potentially harmful (arrhythmias and adverse metabolic sequelae). Prevention of prerenal ARF by careful patient selection and supervision, and rapid response to altered hemodynamic status and oliguria, can help to reduce the amount of dialysis-requiring ATN in hospital.

ATN ARF

Prerenal ARF and ischemic ATN are part of a spectrum of renal responses to renal hypoperfusion. Prevention of contrast nephropathy is best achieved by identification of 'at-risk' subjects (older, diabetic, myeloma, metformin), achievement of adequate hydration and urine output (using 0.45% or 0.9% saline intravenously), and possibly by N-acetyl cysteine for 48 hours before and after contrast. Reducing the amount of injected contrast to the bare minimum in 'at-risk' cases is sensible. Some drug toxicities can be avoided, especially where concentrations can be measured (lithium, gentamicin, vancomycin), hydration ensured (aciclovir [acyclovir]), or less nephrotoxic variants used (e.g. lipid-soluble amphotericin).

There is as yet no widely-accepted specific treatment of established ATN (but no shortage of claims for nephroprotective/renal tubular regenerating compounds).

COMPLICATIONS OF ATN ARF

Euvolemia is hard to maintain in this setting, and most patients become severely salt and water overloaded. Loop diuretics (intravenously in difficult cases or where plasma albumin is low, thereby increasing gut edema and reducing drug absorption) with or without thiazides are the mainstay of therapy. *Hyponatremia* is common as free water excretion in ATN is impaired. Careful fluid replacement (intravenous or nasogastric/feed) can prevent or overcome this. *Hyperkalemia* is very common in ARF; in noncatabolic patients plasma potassium rises by 0.5 mmol/day, and can rise by five times this in very catabolic patients or patients with a large amount of damaged tissue (e.g. rhabdomyolysis). Potassium supplements and retaining-drugs must obviously be stopped. Dietary/feeding advice is important. In mild cases calcium resonium by mouth or rectum can be effective in the short term. If there is urine being produced, loop diuretics are kaliuretic. More severe cases required insulin and dextrose, more rarely hypertonic saline or bicarbonate, with emergency intervention with boluses of 10% calcium gluconate. These bolus maneuvers merely 'hide' potassium in cells, and this strategy is doomed to failure unless the excess potassium is actually excreted from the body. If this is not possible, dialysis is needed.

The use of hypertonic intravenous sodium bicarbonate acutely to correct *acidoses* (diabetic ketoacidotic, lactic, renal failure) has fallen into opprobrium – this relates to the osmolar, sodium, and fluid loads imposed, and the fact that bicarbonate on dissociation is a carbon dioxide donor. Oral sodium bicarbonate is often used slowly to correct mild metabolic acidosis.

Hyperphosphatemia, hypocalcemia, and hyperuricemia are further potential metabolic complications.

Nutrition needs active management during ARF. Catabolism may be net 200 g protein/day. Adequate calories are needed, without excessive protein, sodium, or potassium.

Bleeding is a significant issue in ARF. Sites include gastrointestinal tract, and sites of trauma, line insertion, and operations. Prophylactic measures against peptic ulceration are very sensible (e.g. proton pump inhibitors). Uremia is associated with an acquired platelet functional

Management and outcome (*continued*)

defect (reduced aggregability and reduced activation) which can be measured as a prolonged bleeding time. Dialysis best deals with this, but transfusion to a hemoglobin of >10 g/l (1 g/dl) also helps. Clearly careful thought needs to be given to the continued use of antiplatelet agents and other anticoagulants in ARF. Uremic bleeding can be treated with 1-deamino-8-D-arginine vasopressin (an analogue of ADH) which transiently releases endogenous endothelial cell stores of factor VIII–von Willebrand factor complexes; these increase platelet adhesion to the vessel wall. The effect of this intervention is rapid (within minutes) but wanes rapidly and there is tachyphylaxis. Cryoprecipitate can also be helpful, but takes 8–24 hours to work.

DIALYSIS IN ARF

The absolute indications for dialysis are the development of the uremic syndrome or irremediable and life-threatening hyperkalemia (**275–277**), acidosis, or pulmonary edema (**278**). If recovery is not imminent, most nephrologists would commence dialysis with a plasma creatinine >7.0 mg/dl (619 μmol/l). If the patient is not in a medical facility where some sort of dialysis is available, the patient needs to be made safe to transfer to a suitable facility; in practice hyperkalemia and pulmonary edema are the two risks for sudden deterioration. Emergency hemofiltration on the ICU at a referring hospital is safer than a long risky journey with a hypoxic hyperkalemic patient.

What type of renal replacement therapy to institute depends in part on local factors such as facilities and expertise. The options include peritoneal dialysis, intermittent hemodialysis, and continuous therapies. There is evidence though that continuous convective-based therapies are superior (in outcome terms) for sepsis- and ischemia-induced ATN; in part this is due to better removal of circulating cytokines, and also because of the avoidance of further hemodynamic instability that can be seen when using intermittent hemodialysis in an acutely unwell patient.

INTERMITTENT HD

This is performed 3–5 times a week, depending on the fluid removal and catabolism issues. Vascular access is by means of a cuffed double-lumen catheter in a great vein. Use of a biocompatible membrane (e.g. polysulfone, polycarbonate, polyamide, polyacrilonitrile) is associated with a better ARF recovery rate. Dialysate needs to have a bicarbonate-based buffering system. Anticoagulation should be minimized to low-dose heparin, or heparin-free dialysis should be attempted (high flow, saline flushes).

CONTINUOUS HEMOFILTRATION/DIAFILTRATION

Many of the sickest patients with ARF, e.g. those with several organ failure, are hemodynamically unstable and hypercatabolic. Attempts to use intermittent HD usually result in circulatory collapse. It is much preferable to use continuous convective-based renal replacement therapies in this setting. Continuous venovenous filtration (CVVH) and continuous arteriovenous filtration (CAVH) rely on convective clearance of solute across a porous dialysis membrane with fluid replacement with physiologic solutions. Diffusive and convective clearance can usefully be combined in CVVHDF (**279**). Bicarbonate-based buffers are used in severe catabolism or liver failure. In all of these techniques one has the potential to control fluid balance, plasma ionic composition, and remove toxins with as little hemodynamic disturbance as possible.

PERITONEAL DIALYSIS

This is a useful therapy for children and adults where more expensive therapies (see above) are not provided. Although 'gentle' this therapy is very limited in its applicability to a septic unwell patient, and there are risks from the insertion of the peritoneal catheter (as, to be fair, there are for venous access). Peritonitis is another risk (and again, vascular catheter-related sepsis is a major problem in ICU).

OUTCOME IN ARF

The mortality of ARF is about 40% – ranging from 10% for uncomplicated easily reversible ATN to 80%+ for ICU-based multiple-organ failure patients. The age and comorbidities of the typical ARF patient may explain this high mortality rate; most deaths are due now to the underlying cause and not the renal failure *per se* (but sometimes due to complications arising from its treatment).

Patients who survive an ARF episode generally recover sufficiently to live a normal life span. ARF can be irreversible, or only partly reversible, in the elderly with pre-existing renal damage.

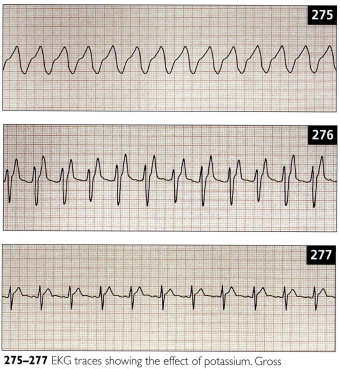

275–277 EKG traces showing the effect of potassium. Gross conduction defects (**275**) due to hyperkalemia (potassium 8.6 mmol/l [mEq/l]). Emergency treatment with 10 ml intravenous 10% calcium gluconate allowed dialysis to start. Tall peaked T-waves (**276**) and some QRS prolongation (potassium 6.6 mmol/l [mEq/l]). After 4 hours' dialysis a normal EKG tracing (**277**) with plasma potassium of 4.0 mmol/l (mEq/l).

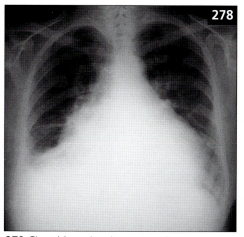

278 Chest X-ray showing acute pulmonary edema which required emergency hemodialysis.

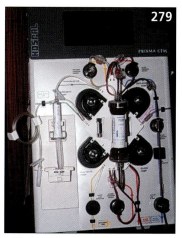

279 Continuous hemofiltration machine.

Chapter Eleven

Chronic renal failure and dialysis

- **Introduction**

- **Natural history**

- **Symptoms, signs, and clinical evaluation**

- **Reversible causes**

- **Complications and consequences**

- **Clinical interventions to retard progression to end-stage renal failure**

- **Dialysis (renal replacement therapy – RRT)**

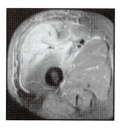 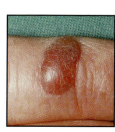 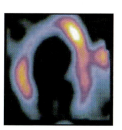 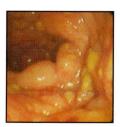

Introduction

The progression of chronic renal failure (CRF) leads in time to end-stage renal failure, at which stage renal replacement therapies (dialysis) need to be considered. In the UK about 110 patients per million population are currently accepted for dialysis each year (i.e. about 5500–6000 patients); this compares with 270 patients per million in the USA in 1996. The incidence of CRF rises very steeply with age, and is much greater in African-American or Asian populations than in Caucasians. The prevalence of patients with significantly elevated plasma creatinine values cannot precisely be estimated, but it might be 2000–3000 per million population. Only a minority of these patients will have seen, or be under the active management of, a nephrologist. Many of the complications that dialysis patients suffer have their origins in the pre-ESRF CRF phase; familiarity with these, and with preventive strategies, mandates a liaison with nephrology specialists. Dialysis patient numbers run at about 5–8 times the incidence; there are about 30,000 dialysis and transplanted patients in the UK and >300,000 in the USA. The UK Renal Registry is beginning to hold epidemiologic and clinical audit data, mirroring the efforts of the United States Renal Data Service (USRDS).

Although in absolute terms the numbers of patients with severe CRF going onto dialysis are modest (especially compared to cardiac or cancer patients), there is a disproportionate financial cost – a typical dialysis patient's health care will 'cost' at least £20,000 (US $30,000) per annum to deliver. Presently 30–40% of all new dialysis patients have diabetes as the underlying causative factor for CRF. As populations have grown more obese, there has been a huge increase in type II diabetes and its attendant complications. Such patients, if they live to enter a dialysis programme, are typically 60–70 years of age, with cardiovascular morbidities, and are very rarely suitable for renal transplantation. Thus only about one in four current dialysis patients can hope to receive a renal transplant.

Natural history

Renal functional decline can often be found to be a linear event when plotted as reciprocal creatinine versus time. Variations around this linearity are, though, common, e.g. intercurrent illnesses, dehydration, drugs. The rate of renal functional decline depends on many factors – these include the etiology of the underlying nephropathy, the quality of blood pressure control, and factors specific to individual patients. Chronic glomerulonephritis causes a faster decline in renal function than is seen in chronic interstitial nephritis.

Various factors affect the progression of CRF. Age is relevant as the incidence of ARF and CRF rises steeply with age. The etiology of CRF is very different for aged patients (hypertension, type 2 diabetes, renovascular and prostatic diseases). Male gender has long been known to be a risk factor for a more rapid decline in renal function; renal diseases are also more common in males. Race is also an important risk factor for CRF, in part because diabetes and hypertension are more common in African-Americans and Asians. There are clearly many genetic factors in the susceptibility to nephropathy (e.g. ACE genotype, aldose reductase, TGF-beta); diabetic and nondiabetic nephropathies cluster in families. Proteinuria is emerging as a prime risk factor for renal decline (and also for cardiovascular mortality in hypertensive and diabetic populations). The Modification of Diet in Renal Disease (MDRD) study shows baseline proteinuria is a strong predictor of future renal decline. Increasing evidence is also incriminating dyslipidemia.

The strongest association of all, however, between a risk factor for nephropathy and a prime mover in renal functional decline, is hypertension and renal disease. The rate of functional decline can vary 10-fold depending on prevalent blood pressure levels. The MDRD study showed the great relevance of blood pressure to renal functional decline in the presence of significant proteinuria (>3 g/24 h). There is clear evidence that smoking cigarettes contributes to adverse renal outcomes.

MECHANISMS OF CRF PROGRESSION

Much information has been derived from a variety of animal models of human uremia. These include 5/6 nephrectomy, puromycin nephropathy, and mercuric chloride nephropathy. The progression of CRF is associated with a stereotyped renal structural reponse, as the kidney has a limited repertoire of reponses to diverse injurious insults. Progressive sclerosis and fibrosis of the glomeruli – glomerulosclerosis – is a cardinal feature of all chronic renal disease.

Initial glomerular endothelial cell injury is followed by inflammation, endothelial cell proliferation, then fibrosis. The endothelial cells have a phenotypic shift from their constitutive antithrombotic, antiproliferative, and antimitotic functions, to prothrombotic, proliferative, and mitogenic characteristics. A wide variety of cytokines and chemokines has been linked with these fundamental changes. The similarity with endothelial response to injury in an artery, and subsequent atherosclerosis, is telling. How acute glomerular injury then resolves is an issue of the greatest importance; clearly in some situations this resolution is not accompanied by any scarring; in others, scarring is severe.

Tubulointerstitial scarring is an extremely important feature of progressive renal problems. Indeed, the severity of tubulointerstitial scarring correlates much better with renal function, and future renal functional predictions, than does the state of the glomeruli. Once again, there is injury, reponse with inflammation, proliferation of fibroblasts, excessive extracellular matrix deposition (collagen types I and III), and scarring/fibrosis. Angiotensin (Ang) II is an important player in this process – the kidney has most of its angiotensin in the Ang II form (unlike any other organ where Ang I predominates).

Vascular sclerosis is another important feature of the structural changes seen in CRF. Renal arteriolar hyalinosis, in the absence of elevated blood pressure, is an early feature. Hyalinosis of afferent and efferent arterioles is a characteristic of diabetes.

Symptoms, signs, and clinical evaluation

Patients with CRF can present 'gradually' i.e. with modest or no symptoms or with a fully-fledged uremic emergency. Unfortunately, a substantial proportion (about one-third) of patients with CRF only present as they require dialysis (either soon, or immediately). As hypertension and diabetes form about 50–60% of the current reasons for ESRF, this is disturbing.

The consequences of late referral can be severe – the uremic emergency has a significant mortality, and protracted anemia, fluid overload, and hypertension will have damaged the left ventricle. As important, an elective planned start to dialysis means the patient is motivated, educated, and involved in his or her health care; as the care of the dialysis patient is best as a partnership, not a dictatorship, those patients denied the chance for physical and mental planning of their renal replacement therapy tend to fare less well.

Reversible causes

It is very important to hold in mind that, although many CRF etiologies are irreversible (e.g. diabetes, except with pancreatic transplantation), many are eminently reversible, e.g. renal tract obstruction, analgesic nephropathy, lupus, vasculitis, membranous glomerulopathy, amyloidosis (rarely), and renal tuberculosis, familial juvenile hyperuricemic nephropathy. Establishing the cause for CRF is important therefore, and requires a full history, examination, and a battery of laboratory and imaging investigations, culminating in a renal biopsy in many cases (except where the cause is obvious for other reasons or the kidneys too contracted to permit biopsy safely). As it is, many patients enter dialysis programmes without a clear-cut diagnosis, with a bland urinary deposit, small scarred kidneys, and negative auto-antibody screens. Such patients could have had interstitial nephritis, hypertension, glomerulonephritis, renal tuberculosis, or sarcoidosis.

Complications and consequences

CARDIOVASCULAR DISEASE

Cardiovascular disease is 3–5-fold increased in patients with chronic renal failure. Even micro-albuminuria significantly increases cardiovascular risk. The reasons include the high prevalence of diabetes, hypertension, and dyslipidemia, but also less 'conventional' factors such as hyper-homocysteinemia, increased oxidative stress, progressive malnutrition, and 'micro-inflammation'.

ANEMIA

Anemia is very common in CRF (most ADPKD patients are spared this) due to a reduction in circulating erythropoietin and some bone marrow resistance to its action. Human recombinant erythropoietin at about 80–120 IU/kg will restore hemoglobin concentrations (the target level is controversial, but 12–13 g/dl [120–130 g/l] seems ideal). Left ventricular size decreases and function improves in virtually all patients, though BP control may need intensification in about one-quarter of patients.

RENAL BONE DISEASE

Renal bone disease is a composite of high- and low-turnover bone diseases. In uremia there is skeletal resistance to the action of circulating PTH, and often incipient vitamin D deficiency (through loss of tubular 1-alphahydroxylase activity). Early symptoms are very rare, so biochemical and radiologic analysis is required. Control of plasma phosphate (dietary compliance, phosphate binders), correction of metabolic acidosis (using oral sodium bicarbonate), and judicious use of vitamin D analogues (e.g. 1-alfacalcidol in the UK, calcitriol in the USA) are required. Over-enthusiasm however can induce low-turnover bone, with problems of increased fracture rate, and increased soft tissue metastatic calcification. (See later discussion in the context of dialysis patients.)

MALNUTRITION

Malnutrition is too common in CRF especially as renal function deteriorates to GFR levels of 10–20 ml/min. Clues to this problem include low/falling cholesterol and falling plasma albumin and plasma creatinine (reflecting loss of muscle bulk, and capable of misinterpretation as renal functional improvement by the uninitiated). Body weight may not alter much; fluid retention/edema dilute its usefulness. In CRF, patients are told to avoid eating many different foodstuffs (to avoid excess sodium, potassium, calcium, phosphate, protein); too often this results in poor calorie intake. Problems with sodium, potassium, and water balance are typically seen when GFR falls below 15–20 ml/min. A low-salt diet is helpful in preventing fluid overload, e.g. 50 mmol (mEq) sodium/day. Water intake must be modulated too. Potassium excess is seen as the need for dialysis gets greater; hyporeninemic hypoaldosteronism (so called 'type IV' renal tubular acidosis seen typically in type II diabetics), and the use of ACE inhibitors and angiotensin receptor blockers contribute to this problem. Beta-blockers are also associated with hyperkalemia in CRF. CRF patients misdiagnosed with heart failure, and placed on ACE inhibitors, beta-blockers, and spironolactone, are guaranteed to run into potassium problems.

SKIN PROBLEMS

Skin problems include excoriations, xerosis, nodular prurigo (**280**), pseudomyxedamatous scleroderma, diffuse brown pigmentation, 'half-and-half' nails (**281**), and bullous eruptions (**282**) (these are due either to large doses of furosemide [frusemide] as a photosensitivity fixed drug eruption, or more rarely as a result of pseudoporphyria).

ENDOCRINE ABNORMALITIES

Endocrine abnormalities include of course the dysregulation of vitamin D, and lack of erythropoietin. In addition, increased reversed fT3 conversion is seen. Reduced insulin degradation by renal tubules is a feature of a GFR <40 ml/min; this, and decreased calorie intake, may substantially reduce insulin or oral hypoglycemic agent requirements in CRF. Insulin resistance, however, also rises with falling GFR, so the relationship between food intake, fasting insulin, glucose, and glucose-altering medications is complex. Testosterone levels are often low in male dialysis patients; prolactin elevation can contribute to gynecomastia. Erectile dysfunction is common (and helped by sildenafil, testosterone, and erythropoietin). Most female dialysis patients are amenorrheic; pregnancy with advanced CRF or on dialysis is highly unusual and rarely successful (see Chapter 9).

INFECTION RATES AND IMMUNE SYSTEM FUNCTION

Infection rates and immune system function are often abnormal in CRF. Infection is a common cause of death and morbidity. T-cell function is defective, as is neutrophil activity against bacteria. Patients are notoriously hard to immunize.

MALIGNANCY

Malignancy is more common in CRF and on dialysis. Multicystic kidneys are one reason, but increased rates of primary liver and thyroid cancers and lymphoma are reported. The reason may relate to impaired immune surveillance, and T-cell function. One 'advantage' of the relative immunosuppression of uremia is the usual behavior of most lupus and vasculitis cases – it is unusual for such patients on dialysis to suffer full-blown relapses, and the intensity of immunosuppression can safely be reduced.

PSYCHIATRIC PROBLEMS

Psychiatric problems are much more common in CRF and dialysis patients. These range from depression, anxiety, and phobias, to full-blown psychosis. Sympathy, realism, education, and counseling are all important. Rarely formal psychiatric review and therapy are needed. Patients with severe mental illness such as schizophrenia, or with profound personality disorders, are especially challenging to manage on dialysis. Though unusual, where patients are rude and unco-operative with the dialysis team, this leads to dialysis staff (typically health-care assistants and nurses) becoming heavily stressed. Even more rarely, violence can make dialysis very difficult. Lack of understanding, fear, and drug abuse, or undiagnosed physical and mental illnesses, can explain these occurrences in some cases.

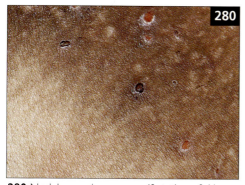

280 Nodular prurigo as a manifestation of skin disorders in chronic renal failure. The skin is diffusely hyperpigmented in areas of intense excoriation.

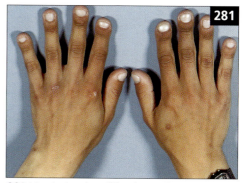

281 Hands showing diffuse lemon-brown pigmentation of chronic uremia, and also showing leuconychia with typical 'half-and-half' nails (proximal pallor, distal pigmentation) of chronic renal failure. Also note gross shortening of distal phalanges (as renal pseudoclubbing – a sign of severe hyperparathyroidism. See **344, 345**).

282 Bulla on a finger (skin photosensitivity reaction to furosemide [frusemide]). Nails also show the proximal pallor and distal rim of pigmentation.

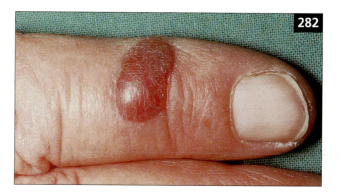

Clinical interventions to retard progression to end-stage renal failure

Dietary manipulation has long been advocated as a means of retarding CRF. Low protein low phosphate diets in 5/6 nephrectomized rats are very effective. The data in human subjects, however, are muddled and confusing. Many trials exist. The largest of them, the MDRD study, followed 840 patients over 3 years and was not able to show a difference in renal functional decline between patients with and without dietary restriction. Re-analysis, and meta-analysis, can provide some suggestions that for severe renal impairment, severe protein restriction can retard GFR decline. However, the practicalities are more complex. First, because of the anorectic effect of uremia, many patients self-restrict their total calorie (and hence protein) intake. Second, there are real dangers in further restricting food intake in patients already proscribed a great deal. Unless there is an intense degree of dietary supervision there is a real danger of inducing malnutrition in a cohort of patients, with attendant risks when these patients reach ESRF.

Blood pressure control by contrast is accepted universally as being of paramount importance. Data from the MRFIT study showed a graded relationship between SBP and DBP and ESRD. The Helsinki Heart Study renal subgroup showed similar findings, with an interaction between BP and lipids. The MDRD study provided further evidence, and suggested that a lower BP target (mean arterial pressure [MAP] 92 mmHg [12.3 kPa]) was more appropriate for patients with heavy (>3 g/24 h) proteinuria than for patients with lesser proteinuria (MAP 98 mmHg [13.1 kPa]). A recent study of polycystic kidney patients, however, could not show a relationship between achieved BP control and future renal functional deterioration.

Recent meta-analyses for the period 1977–99 have suggested that *ACE inhibitors* provide unique nephroprotection, over and above that expected from BP reduction. This is a very controversial area. ACE inhibitors in type 1 diabetic nephropathy, and angiotensin receptor blockers (ARBs) in type 2 diabetic nephropathy, are the gold standard BP reducing agents. In nondiabetic CRF, ACE inhibitors reduce the risk of ESRF by 31% compared to placebo or other BP reducing agents. From the African-American Study, and from the IDNT study, there are now data to suggest that monotherapy with dihydropyridine calcium channel blockers (CCB) are not ideal – these agents cause afferent arteriolar vasodilatation, thus may raise intraglomerular pressure not reduce it,

and are accompanied by little or no reduction in micro-albuminuria/proteinuria. However, CCBs are very effective antihypertensives, and using them in concert with an ACE inhibitor/ARB is highly effective and confers nephroprotection.

It is surprising how often it is forgotten that a 10–15% fall in GFR is often seen on the administration of an ACE inhibitor/ARB. The small and nonprogressive rise in plasma creatinine should be monitored carefully, but is not a reason to withdraw the drugs. Indeed, there is some evidence that patients who show this hemodynamic response fare best in the longer term. Of course, in the presence of severe renal artery stenosis, where glomerular filtration is dependent exclusively on angiotensin II-mediated efferent arteriolar vasoconstriction, the administration of an ACE inhibitor/ARB can lead to a disastrous GFR reduction (Chapter 5). Hyperkalemia after ACE inhibition is seen in about 5–10% of patients with CRF; this is contrasted with about 1–2% with an ARB.

There is growing evidence to support the use of statin-based lipid lowering therapy to help retard progressive renal functional decline, especially in proteinuric renal disease. Finally, careful supervision and follow-up of CRF patients is vital to success – these patients and their generalist physicians must know that they should not take NSAIDs, tetracyclines, or other potentially nephrotoxic drugs.

TRANSITION FROM PREDIALYSIS TO RRT

One of the prime reasons for timely nephrologic referral of a patient with declining renal function is to facilitate an orderly start of renal replacement therapy. Amongst the goals to be achieved in this setting, uppermost are reducing the rate of renal functional decline to a minimum, reversing/preventing the complications of renal disease at this stage (e.g. renal bone disease, anemia, acidosis, left ventricular hypertrophy), formation of dialysis access (e.g. arteriovenous fistula) in good time, and allowing the patient and carers to be educated about renal disease, its implications, and treatments.

There can be no precise creatinine value or GFR at which dialysis must be started. With careful attention to detail many patients can function well even with GFR values <10 ml/min. In certain cases, fluid overload or hyperkalemia mandate a sudden start of RRT. In other cases, loss of appetite/nausea or falling albumin or body weight are signs that dialysis should be started.

Dialysis (renal replacement therapy – RRT)

INTRODUCTION

Hemodialysis (HD) has evolved from decidedly primitive physical arrangements to a computerized, mechanized maneuver. This 'advance' however is not what it seems – the principles of dialysis four decades ago were substantially similar to those in use now. Blood needs to be withdrawn from the circulation in a sterile way without clotting, to bathe one side of a semipermeable membrane, across which counterflows prepprepared dialysate, and then be returned safely to the patient. Cannulae, anticoagulation, sterility, air embolism – all of these were major impedimenta in the early days – now solved by technologic advances. Initially all dialysis was seen as a 'bridge' to renal recovery from injury, or until renal transplantation could take place (rather like a left ventricular assist device might now be viewed). Gradually it was the case that more and more patients were dialysed for longer, and the idea of a chronic RRT service developed. Initially the acceptance criteria for such programmes were both strict and paternalistic. As time has progressed there are fewer bars to providing long-term RRT.

A 16-station hemodialysis unit, operating three shifts/day and 6 days/week dialysing patients thrice-weekly, will perform 15,000 hemodialyses per annum – and >99% of these sessions will take place as scheduled.

Peritoneal dialysis (e.g. CAPD) has had a shorter history (starting 1975) as a chronic RRT. There were, as for HD, many technical problems in its initial use. Long-term technique survival is rarer for CAPD than for HD. Initial survival rates are comparable. In a civilized society, patients should be encouraged to exercise choice about how they dialyse; this helps to involve the patient in his own long-term care. The techniques HD and CAPD are often regrettably seen as mutually exclusive – most patients will require some time on each of these dialysis modalities. Many patients do not have the physical or mental attributes to permit self-dialysis; in these cases, unit-based HD is preferred unless relatives or carers can be trained to do CAPD.

HEMODIALYSIS

Modern HD can take place at home, in a dialysis center away from a main hospital ('satellite dialysis unit') or at a main hospital site (for more medically-dependent patients). Blood access is best achieved using an arteriovenous fistula (**283**); these depend on arterialization of peripheral veins in the upper or lower arm due to exposure of veins to arterial pressure. This process can take 4–8 weeks to occur (and is characterized by marked vessel wall thickening thus permitting large needle (14 or 15 French Guage) insertion. Gortex/PTFE grafts are alternatives. Short- and long-term tunnelled venous catheters, single- or double-lumen, are further alternatives (**284**). Anticoagulation is achieved typically with a bolus and then an infusion of intravenous heparin. Treatment duration is typically for 4 hours, thrice-weekly, with arterial blood flow of 250–300 ml/min and dialysate flow of 500–600 ml/min. The dialysate is bicarbonate-buffered, and potassium, calcium, and magnesium concentrations can be varied.

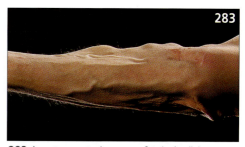

283 A mature arteriovenous fistula (radial anastomosis).

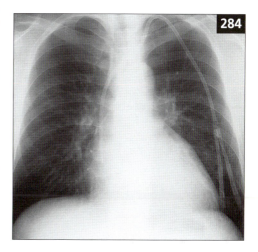

284 Plain chest X-ray showing a tunnelled left internal jugular 'Permcath'.

Dialysis (RRT) (*continued*)

The typical modern dialysis machine (**285**) can vary dialysis bicarbonate, sodium, and dialysate temperature in sophisticated ways.

There is increasing interest in daily HD, with short treatment times (e.g. 2 hours). By this means several significant complications of HD (e.g. hypertension, left ventricular hypertrophy, and hyperphosphatemia) can be avoided.

Complications of acute hemodialysis

There are many complications that can arise because of HD. We shall consider these first as those arising during, or as a direct result of, the hemodialysis session. The other main group of complications is as a result of being on dialysis for some time (and overlaps substantially with complications seen in long-term CAPD patients); this will be discussed at the end of this chapter as a result.

There are various adverse reactions that can occur as a result of the passage of patients' blood over the surface components of the extracorporeal circuit. These can be grouped by time of onset:

Immediate (i.e. within the first 30 minutes)

Anaphylaxis is rare, mediated by IgE, and reflects exposure of blood to ethylene oxide, glutaraldehyde, or renalin (used in sterilizing dialysers). Treatment involves stopping HD, avoiding blood return to the patient, and any/all of antihistamines, corticosteroids, and epinephrine (adrenaline). Alternative sterilization techniques (e.g. irradiation), and increased predialysis dialyser flushing, are helpful.

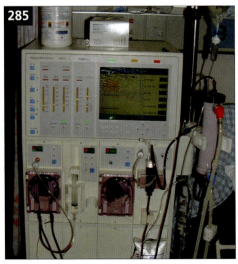

285 A typical modern hemodialysis machine.

Similar reactions in patients on ACE inhibitors using AN69 membranes have been recorded (due to bradykinin release).

Iron dextran infusions can also induce anaphylactoid reactions on dialysis.

Early (30–60 minutes)

This is a mild reaction, with fever due to activation of white cells and platelets by the dialysis membrane. This was more often seen with so-called bioincompatible dialysis membranes (e.g. cuprophane), which have largely been superseded by more expensive biocompatible materials.

Any time

Pyrogen reactions are due to contamination of dialysis fluid by bacteria or bacterial endotoxins. The very highest standards of water preparation (ionic and microbiologic) are mandatory (but expensive).

HEMODYNAMIC COMPLICATIONS

The next group of complications arises from the hemodynamic effects that dialysis has, and the circulatory response mediated by baroreceptors and the autonomic and sympathetic nervous systems.

Dialysis hypotension

Symptomatic intradialytic hypotension occurs in 10–30% of dialysis treatments. It can shorten dialysis times, result in hypertension as a consequence of maneuvers to avoid hypotension, and may possibly have deleterious effects on brain and cardiac perfusion if severe, prolonged, or repeated.

The etiopathogenesis is complex and multifactorial – including autonomic neuropathy, antihypertensive medications, sepsis, bloodpooling, increased body core temperature, hypoalbuminemia, and anemia. Acetate-buffered dialysis (rare in the developed world), and low sodium and calcium dialysate concentrations, also are risk factors.

Treatment is by temporary cessation of dialysis, reverse Trendelenburg position, and by saline infusions. Prevention is by attending to as many risk factors as possible. Sodium profiling, cooled dialysate, and on-line biofeedback ultrafiltration monitoring may all help. Midodrine (an alpha-agonist) has also been successfully used.

Dialysis hypertension

BP control in dialysis patients is rarely optimal or optimizable. Large doses of several antihypertensives may control BP to a degree between dialysis sessions, but brings with it a large risk of intradialytic BP instability. Many patients show clear volume dependency in their BP. In others the relationship is more subtle. Increased sympathetic drive, accumulation of pressor compounds, defective nitric oxide synthase/ endogenous inhibitors of nitric oxide synthase (e.g. asymmetric dimethylarginine [ADMA]), and erythropoietin are other reasons for dialysis patients to be hypertensive. Diurnal BP rhythm is generally very deranged in dialysis patients, with many showing a rise in BP with recumbency (**286**). Autonomic dysfunction is likely to be a major reason for this, which has prognostic implications. For many patients, the price paid for short dialysis sessions and excessive sodium dialysate concentrations (which engineer some cardiovascular stability), is chronic salt and water overload, and chronic refractory hypertension. It has been known for 40 years that long, slow dialysis, or, more recently, daily dialysis, can normalize BP without the use of antihypertensives. Some patients show a vigorous end-of-dialysis BP surge – this is as a result of hypokalemia/hypovolemia stimulation of an intact renin–angiotensin system. This can be blocked by angiotensin antagonists.

Arrhythmias and sudden death
Sudden death rates (more often after than before or during HD) are vastly increased in dialysis patients (mainly but not exclusively HD). This is especially the case for type 1 diabetics on HD. Eighty per cent of these sudden deaths are as a result of ventricular fibrillation. End-of-dialysis hypokalemia, hypocalcemia, and hypomagnesemia, and mild intradialytic hypoxemia are partly to blame, as are malignant ventricular re-entrant arrythmias resulting from a combination of coronary artery disease, inter-cardiomyocyte fibrosis seen in the uremic myocardium, and from left ventricular hypertrophy. Pericarditis and conducting system calcification are also responsible for arrhythmias on dialysis. Prevention is by scrupulous attention to postdialysis electrolyte concentrations, by avoiding digoxin use where possible, and by prompt diagnosis and treatment of ischemic heart disease.

MISCELLANEOUS COMPLICATIONS
Neuromuscular complications
Up to 25% of patients can report muscle cramps, usually in the legs, towards the end of dialysis – this seems to be related to incipient or real hypovolemia, and also low calcium and magnesium concentrations. Quinine, diazepam, and less aggressive dialysis schedules may relieve the symptoms, which, when severe, are a cause of premature dialysis session discontinuation.

Restless legs can occur on dialysis, or between sessions. The legs either twitch (myoclonus) or the patient experiences an irresistible desire to move their legs because of dysesthesiae. Co-existing iron deficiency anemia and vascular insufficiency may exacerbate these problems. Clonazepam, phenytoin, L-DOPA and gabapentin may all help.

Dialysis disequilibration syndrome is fortunately rare. Risk factors are more aggressive dialysis techniques (greater solute removal per unit time) and intercurrent illnesses. Restlessness, agitation, headache, nausea, vomiting, blurred vision, seizures, and coma are seen. It may result from transient osmotic disquilibrium in neurons; cerebral imaging shows cerebral edema. When mild the syndrome is rapidly reversible. Short, gentle dialysis sessions minimize risk.

Seizures are rare on dialysis – their causation is multifactorial, including hypoxia, hypertension, disequilibrium, metabolic (low calcium, magnesium, blood glucose), or removal of anticonvulsants by HD.

Technical mishaps and disasters
Over the 40 years of regular HD many different catastrophes have been recorded. Only the more common are described.

Hemorrhage/circuit blood loss is still a feared but very rare occurrence: large bore needles in arterialized veins, with a uremic platelet defect, and systemic anticoagulation +/- antiplatelet drugs are the reasons. Dialysis machines respond to a fall in pressure (such as occurs with hemorrhage) by automatically ceasing dialysis and by sounding alarms.

Air embolism (split lines, or bubble formation) can be lethal. Clinical manifestations

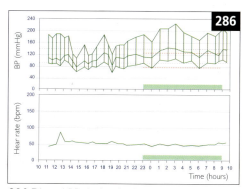

286 Diurnal BP rhythm is abnormal in uremia – in this tracing it can clearly be seen that BP rises during the sleep period (marked by the green hatched area on the BP tracing).

Dialysis (RRT) (*continued*)

depend on the amount of air, how it is introduced, how quickly, and the patient's position. Emboli in the cerebral circulation can be manifest as seizure and coma. Air in the right ventricle causes cardiovascular collapse. Initial management is to clamp all lines, stop the pumps, and place the patient in the left Trendelenburg position, followed by oxygen, intubation and ventilation. Air can be aspirated from the right ventricle.

Incorrect dialysate composition is rare but possible, as the only practical safeguard is dialysate electrical conductivity monitoring. Thus deviations in dialysate sodium will be picked up, but not bicarbonate or calcium problems. Hyponatremia, hypernatremia, hypocalcemia, hypercalcemia, metabolic acidosis, and alkalosis can all be manufactured by faulty dialysis circuits.

Access-related problems

Arteriovenous fistulae are robust and by far the most reliable form of dialysis access. Infection is rare. Stenosis at the site of arteriovenous anastomosis can occur early, and prevent maturation (angioplasty may help this). Other typical sites for fistula stenosis relate to needle-sites, or previous central vein cannulation. Clues to the presence of stenoses include local aneurysmal dilatation (**287**), increasing venous pressure, and reduced dialysis solute clearances. Angioplasty can resolve these difficulties (**288, 289**). ACE inhibition may reduce the tendency to fistula stenosis; poor calcium–phosphate control may contribute to it. Fistula occlusion by thrombosis rarely occurs except when there are adverse factors such as hypercoagulability, low blood pressure, or flow, e.g. with a severe stenosis. A good fistula can provide excellent dialysis for two decades. Central venous lines are a poor (but in some patients necessary) substitute for a fistula. Infection and thrombosis are the chief complications. The presence of the line can cause stenosis/thrombosis of central veins (**290–294**).

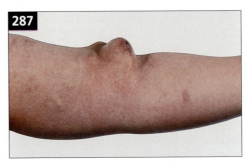

287 Local aneurysmal dilatation of an arteriovenous fistula due to an upper arm fistula stenosis.

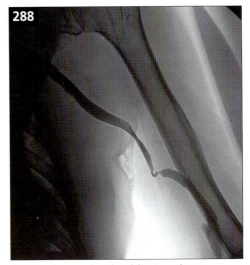

288 Angiogram showing tight stenosis at a needling site of an AVF.

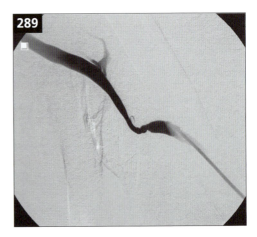

289 Angiogram showing the result of balloon angioplasty – an improved appearance. Blood flows were higher, venous pressures lower, and dialysis clearances improved. These problems though can recur and require repeated treatment or stenting/operative revision.

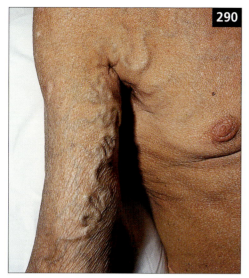

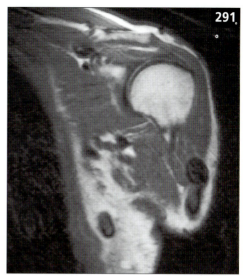

290 Distended veins on the surface of the upper arm and chest herald central venous obstruction and collateral formation.

291 An MR image of the shoulder showing huge collateral venous channels.

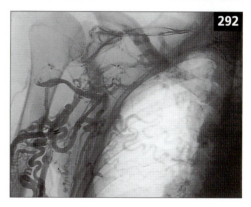

292 A venogram for the patient shown in (290) revealing central venous obstruction and multiple collateral channels.

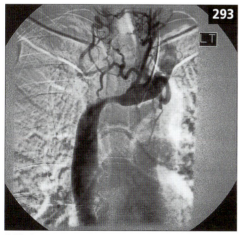

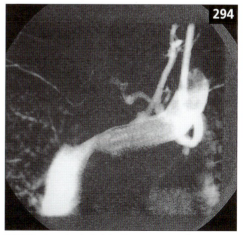

293 Angiogram showing a severe stenosis of the innominate vein secondary to long-term use of a central venous dialysis catheter for dialysis.

294 Post angioplasty/stent appearance for venous stenosis shown in (293).

Dialysis (RRT) (*continued*)

Rarely, a right atrial thrombus can form (**295**) on long-term cannula that enter the right atrium (which can lead to sepsis/pulmonary emboli). Incorrect cannula placement can be life-threatening (**296, 297**).

PERITONEAL DIALYSIS

The peritoneal membrane is semi-permeable and therefore permits dialysis if a sterile dialysate is placed into the abdominal cavity. Some solute is also removed by convection and by solute drag. Transport across the peritoneal membrane is linked to vascular surface area and to intrinsic peritoneal permeability.

There are many different designs of peritoneal catheter now available. There are usually one or two cuffs to provoke subcutaneous fibrosis (helping to anchor the catheter and to reduce the risk of infection tracking back alongside the catheter). Insertion methods vary from direct vision under general anesthesia, to 'blind' insertion using the Seldinger technique in a conscious patient. The latter method results in a greater complication rate, including hematoma formation (**298**) or perforation of abdominal viscera.

Peritoneal dialysis (PD) involves filling the abdominal cavity with dialysis fluid, allowing this fluid to 'dwell' for a while, then draining it out to be replaced with fresh dialysate. This takes place (as CAPD) typically using 2–2.5 liter volumes, four to five times daily, 7 days a week. Machines can perform overnight dialysis using a rapid sequence of exchanges (automated peritoneal dialysis, APD).

All PD fluids contain sodium, calcium, magnesium, and chloride. Lactate is the usual buffer (recently bicarbonate bags with two/three chambers have been developed). The osmotic agent is glucose – all PD fluid is grossly hyperosmolar, and, at pH 5.2, hardly physiological. Other fluids are now available, e.g. a glucose polymer Icodextrin as a 7.5% solution which works by colloid osmosis, and a 1.1% amino acid mixture.

To check that enough solute clearance is taking place a 24-hour collection of spent dialysate can be undertaken. Also a peritoneal equilibration test can be performed (using 2.27% glucose dwelling for 4 hours). Results are expressed as the ratio of dialysate to plasma creatinine. Ultrafiltration (water removal) can be assessed by examining the patients' daily records, including body weights. Residual renal function is important to assess; indeed, for many patients, the gradual loss of residual renal function over time on dialysis eventually undermines their ability to continue with peritoneal dialysis.

How much PD is 'necessary' is a vexed question not completely answered by trials. The recent CANUSA trial (suggesting that achieving and maintaining as much solute clearance as possible is best) seems to have been contradicted by a larger Mexican (ADEMEX) trial. Increasing solute clearance can be brought about by increasing the number, or volume, of exchanges – at the expense of quality of life and an increased risk of complications. As residual renal function declines, patients can experience progressive problems maintaining fluid balance, BP control, and adequate solute clearance – in part because with time and constant exposure to unphysiologic solutions, the peritoneal membrane structure changes and function deteriorates. Anuric patients are challenging to maintain long-term on PD.

There are many complications that arise as a result of continued PD. These can be classified into infectious and noninfectious.

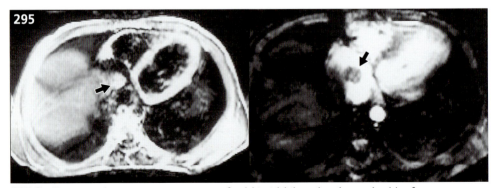

295 Cardiac magnetic resonance appearance of a right atrial thrombus (arrows) arising from a dialysis cannula.

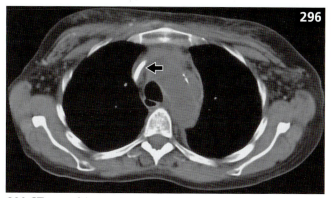

296 CT scan of thorax showing a dialysis cannula (arrow) traversing the mediastinum and peri-aortic hematoma.

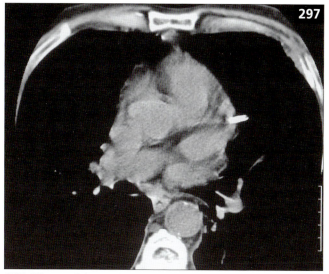

297 CT scan of thorax showing a dialysis cannula traversing the mediastinum. The tip is in the pericardial space.

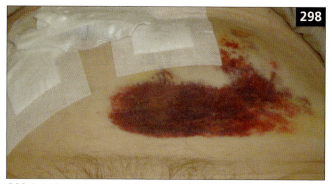

298 Anterior abdominal wall hematoma after peritoneal dialysis cannula insertion.

Dialysis (RRT) (*continued*)

INFECTIOUS COMPLICATIONS

Without doubt the most important complication of PD is infection in the peritoneal cavity. Infection can be virtually asymptomatic or cause severe systemic upset. Usually colicky abdominal pain and cloudy effluent (white cell content of >100 white cells/mm^3 (10^8/l) [**299**]) are the clues. Fever and raised CRP are typical. Empirical antibiotics are started (as either intravenous or intraperitoneal boluses, then added to the bags) and then changed as appropriate once PD fluid cultures have been analyzed. The commonest infection is with *Staphylococcus* spp. Culture of a mixed growth, particularly Gram-negatives and anerobes, strongly suggests abdominal viscus perforation or abscess. Failure to respond to antibiotics is an indication for catheter removal +/- laparotomy. Fungal infections, though rare, invariably require catheter removal for recovery (**300**). Sterile peritonitis,

eosinophilic or not, is rarely seen, and should not constitute >10% of all peritonitis episodes – it is a composite of chemical irritation, drug/fluid allergic reaction, and failure to culture micro-organisms with fastitidious growth requirements. In a well-run unit, infection rates of about 1–2 per 24 patient therapy months should be expected. Repeated cycles of peritoneal infection can damage peritoneal membrane structure irreparably. Persistent fever and raised inflammatory markers for many days or weeks after a severe peritonitis episode should alert the nephrologist to the possibilities of localized infected collections in the abdomen (**301**), peritoneal tuberculosis, or sclerosing peritonitis (see below).

Infection of the exit site or subcutaneous catheter tunnel (**302, 303**) are serious and in time can lead to peritonitis. Topical (and nasal) treatments can help eradication and prevent reinfection. Systemic antibiotics are often required, and refractory cases require catheter removal.

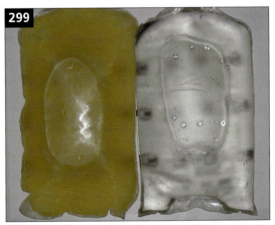

299 PD fluid is normally perfectly clear (PD bag right of picture). In peritonitis the fluid becomes turbid (left of picture) due to white blood cells and fibrin.

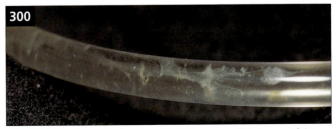

300 Fungal hyphae growing along the PD cannula. This is one of the later signs of fungal peritonitis. It is virtually impossible to eradicate fungal infections without cannula removal.

301 After some episodes of severe peritonitis, especially if the PD cannula is removed without a laparotomy and wash-out, residual 'puddles' of infected PD fluid remain and can form infected collections/abscesses. CT scan of the abdomen showing an anterior abdominal wall infected collection (arrow) that required percutaneous drainage and prolonged antibiotics.

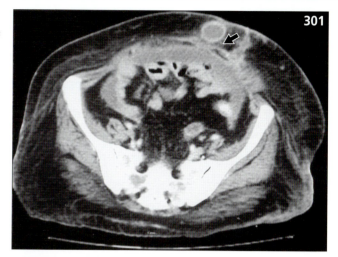

302 There was an associated leak of peritoneal dialysis fluid (as shown by the contouring of the anterior abdominal wall in this thin patient [see **304, 305**]).

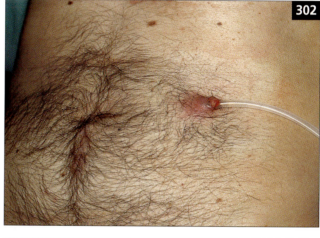

303 Red swollen 'exit-site' where the cannula emerges from its long subcutaneous tunnel. This was due to *Pseudomonas aeruginosa* infection. The redness extends along the proximal part of the tunnel (so this was also a tunnel infection).

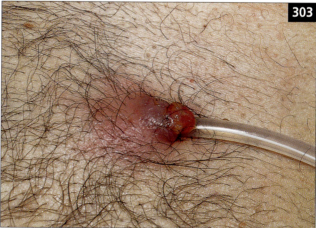

Dialysis (RRT) (*continued*)

NONINFECTIOUS COMPLICATIONS

Catheter migration/omental capture can mean the end of the catheter is enmeshed in exuberant omentum, preventing drainage. Re-implantation and omentectomy are helpful. Constipation (very common on PD) can cause catheter displacement (**304, 305**).

A peritoneal leak (**306, 307**) can occur early after insertion of the catheter if healing is delayed, or intra-abdominal pressure high. Treatment is by resting from PD, or the use of very small exchange volumes. Refractory cases will need surgical repair with a mesh. Herniae are common with longer-term PD, polycystic kidney disease, and large exchange volumes. Again, repair is needed, and recurrences are common. Fluid can escape across the diaphragm to cause hydrothorax.

Failure of ultrafiltration can occur when the osmotic (glucose) gradient collapses (type I failure) – use of shorter exchange dwell times, or an alternative osmotic agent (icodextrin) help. Type II failure occurs with a structural change in the peritoneum – sclerosing (encapsulating) peritonitis is a very serious complication. The peritoneal membrane becomes very thickened, with loss of ultrafiltration and small solute clearance typical. This happens to about 20% of patients continuously exposed to PD solutions for 8 years or more (and to 50% of those on PD for >12 years). It can be triggered by peritonitis or after a series of severe peritonitis episodes. Reactions to acetate, to chlorhexidine and, probably, to glucose degradation products (formed in the manufacture of PD fluid) are likely causes. In some cases the peritoneal membrane becomes grossly thickened and starts to 'invade' the bowel wall (**308–316**). This causes nausea, vomiting, small bowel obstruction, malabsorption, and death. Careful enteroclysis may help, as may TPN and immunosuppressive drugs (prednisolone and azathioprine). Transplantation is the definitive therapy.

An aggressive calcific sclerosing peritonitis can occur with a bloody effluent, abdominal pain and calcified bowel loops grinding against one another with peristalsis (**317–319**).

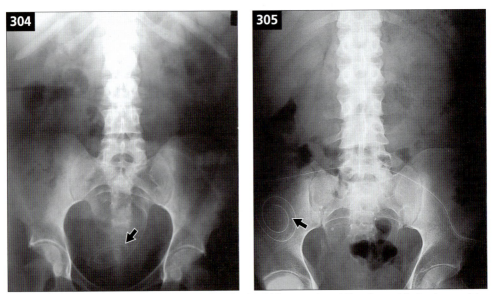

304, 305 The tip of the peritoneal dialysis cannula should lie near the midline (arrow) in the true pelvis (**304**). In this case (**305**) it is grossly displaced to the right (arrow) and superior to where it should lie. Erratic and poor drianage of PD fluid is what the patient notices. In this case severe constipation has caused the migration, which can be treated. Omental capture, another cause of catheter malposition, requires exploration, omentectomy, and resuturing of the catheter in its correct position.

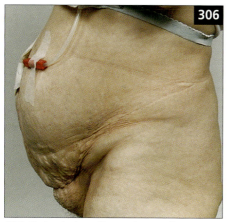

306 Abdominal swelling, and peau d'orange appearance of skin in a subcutaneous leak of PD fluid.

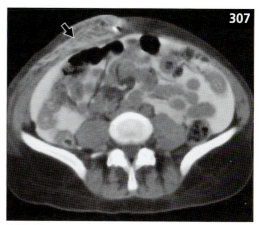

307 CT scan appearance of a subcutaneous leak of PD fluid (arrow).

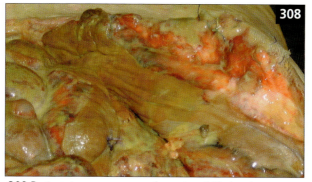

308 Postmortem appearance of grossly wrinkled and thickened parietal peritoneum in a case of sclerosing encapsulating peritonitis.

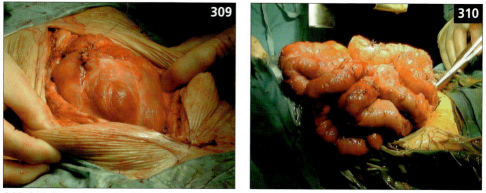

309, 310 Sclerosing peritonitis at laparotomy. Initial site once peritoneum incised (**309**): instead of peritoneal space and free bowel loops, a large inflammatory pannus is present which completely binds together all bowel loops. No anatomic planes for dissection are visible. **310** After 6 hours' painstaking dissection, and many inevitable serosal lesions and some full thickness bowel perforations, the small bowel has been dissected out and freed from the fibrosis.

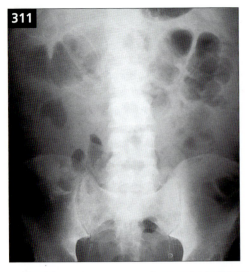

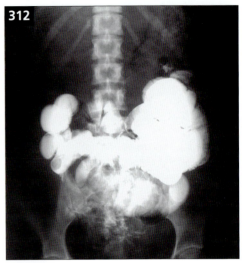

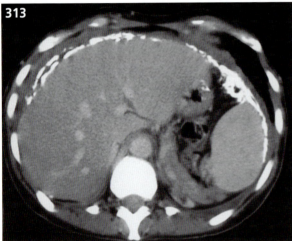

311, 312 Plain X-ray (**311**) of the abdomen showing linear peritoneal calcification, heralding sclerosing peritonitis, often most visible in the pelvis. Dilated small bowel loops are visible too. Barium study (**312**): 24 hours after ingesting barium there is stasis in the mid-small bowel, no barium in the pelvis, but intense pelvic calcification.

313 CT scan of the abdomen in a case of sclerosing encapsulating peritonitis. Thickened parietal peritoneum is visible (with many areas of calcification), particularly intense around the spleen.

314 The small bowel loops are focally dilated and thick-walled/matted together centrally due to the multiple adhesions. There is plentiful ascites (the patient was no longer on peritoneal dialysis).

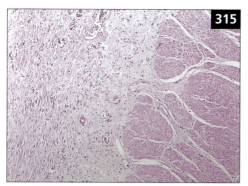

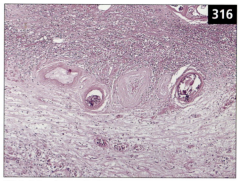

315 The strands of fibrous tissue 'invade' the muscularis mucosa of the large bowel leading to atony/obstruction (H+E ×100).

316 Histology of sclerosing encapsulating peritonitis. Thickened peritoneum, a band of amorphous fibrous tissue, and diabetiform changes in the peritoneal blood vessels are seen (H+E ×250).

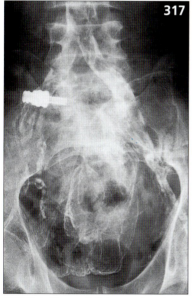

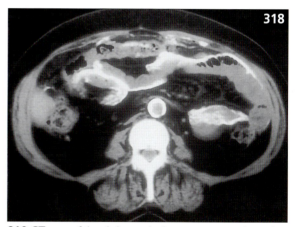

318 CT scan of the abdomen in the same case as shown in **311, 312**. Heavy calcification is present on the antimesenteric border of many small bowel loops.

317 Plain X-ray of abdomen showing remarkable series of curvilinear calcifications in a case of calcific sclerosing peritonitis.

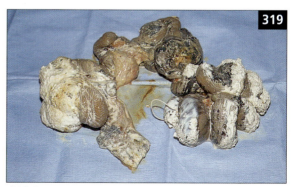

319 Postmortem appearance of intense calcification on the antimesenteric side of small bowel loops, giving rise to the CT scan appearances in **313, 314**.

Dialysis (RRT) (*continued*)

LONGER-TERM COMPLICATIONS OF (ALL) DIALYSIS

There are inevitable consequences of relying on renal replacement therapy for a protracted period. In the simplest terms, expected life-span is much reduced – someone aged 20 years starting dialysis can expect at most 20–25 more years of life on dialysis; someone starting dialysis aged 70 years can expect only 4–6 years. As a rule of thumb, patients can only expect 50% of the actuarially-calculated life-span remaining, and much less than even this if there are significant co-morbidities at the time dialysis begins, e.g. active ischemic heart disease.

Coronary artery disease (CAD)

CAD is much more prevalent in dialysis patients. The prevalence varies from 10–15% in young subjects to >80% of type 1 diabetics over 50 years of age. The risk factors are similar to the non-uremic population, with smoking exerting a particularly malign influence. Symptoms are often more subtle, or absent, due to a more sedentary life-style, and autonomic neuropathy. Screening procedures (EKG, stress-EKG, biochemical markers, e.g. troponin-I, troponin-T, soluble FAS, nuclear scintigraphy [320], electron-beam CT scanning [321]) are all of some use, but their specificity and sensitivity are both significantly less than is the case for nonuremic cohorts. Thus coronary angiography (322) is often the only way effectively to screen for the presence of significant CAD. CAD in uremia is often more distal, more calcified, and more diffuse – all of these features make interventions more complex and less likely

to succeed. Coronary artery angioplasty, rotational atherectomy, followed by stenting (perhaps using stents impregnated with the immuno-modulatory drug sirolimus) are effective maneuvers in experienced centers. The mortality and morbidity from CABG is greater (by about 3–5-fold) than is the case for nonuremic subjects – but if successful the long-term results are much better than, e.g. for coronary angioplasty (where recurrence rates of 80% have been reported at 12 months). Peripheral vascular disease (small vessel, heavily-calcified, 'diabetiform' in behavior) is also a problem seen with increased exposure to dialysis. The calcification, both medial and intimal, once again reduces the effectiveness of angioplasty, and significantly increases the risks of attempted reconstructive arterial surgery.

Ectopic calcification

The vascular calcification referred to above is an example of a very widespread problem for dialysis patients, namely ectopic calcification, which we are now seeing with increased frequency. The etiology is complex and reflects, first, elevated calcium–phosphate product; second, the reduced buffering capacity of the skeleton (which can be due to leaching out of calcium and phosphate by PTH in hyperparathyoidism exacerbated by excess use of vitamin D analogues, and also where overuse of calcium salts and vitamin D analogues have produced a low-turnover bone state); and, finally, the absence of a renal route of excretion of excess calcium and phosphate. Calcification can take place in skin (and be a cause of nodular prurigo), in the joints as peri-articular tumoral masses (323) giving rise to pain, immobility, joint hemorrhage, and infection), in the lungs and

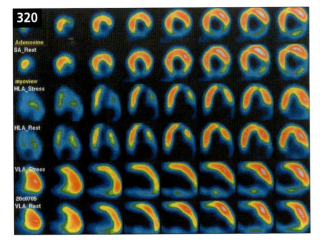

320 Adenosine-myoview scan of the myocardial blood flow patterns in an asymptomatic diabetic dialysis patient being investigated for potential transplantation. The resting scan shows normal blood distribution, but after adenosine (a vasodilator) is injected there is reduced blood flow to the anterior wall of the left ventricle, indicating obstructive coronary artery disease in the left coronary artery.

321 An electron-beam (ultrafast) CT scan of the heart of a long-term dialysis patient showing gross calcification of the left coronary artery.

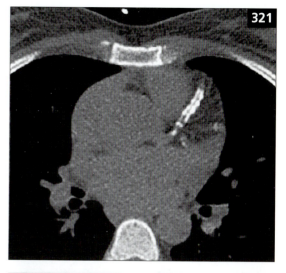

322 A coronary angiogram showing a tight proximal stenosis of the left anterior descending coronary artery.

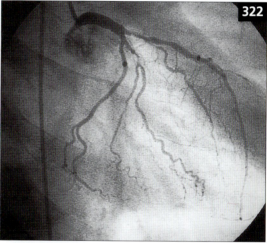

323 X-ray of right shoulder showing a huge 'tumoral' calcific mass (arrow) in/around the shoulder joint.

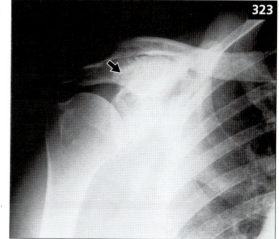

Dialysis (RRT) (*continued*)

myocardium giving rise to dyspnea, respiratory failure, LV dysfunction and conduction defects (**324**), and in the great arteries – aorta (**325, 326**), iliacs (**327**), and smaller, e.g. digital arteries (**328, 329**). The calcification is, as in diabetes, in the medial layer of the vessel wall (like Monkeberg's medial sclerosis, as in **328, 329**), but calcification can also be abluminal and intimal, which is where most vascular calcification is seen in nonuremic subjects, i.e. as part of complex/mature atheroma. Atheroma is calcified much more early and to a greater extent than in nonuremic subjects. Ectopic calcification can also affect the aortic and mitral valves, leading to stenosis, regurgitation, and endocarditis (**330, 331**). The commonest organism responsible for endocarditis in dialysis patients is *Staphylococcus aureus* (mortality is greatly in excess of 50%).

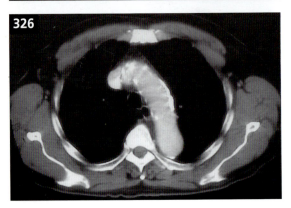

324 Diffuse myocardial calcification (shown post mortem).

325 Aortic calcification. Thoracic CT scan showing several discrete patches of aortic arch wall calcification in a dialysis patient.

326 Abdominal CT scan of the same patient as **325** showing heavy concentric aortic wall calcification.

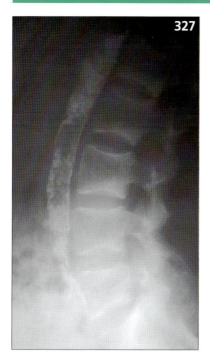

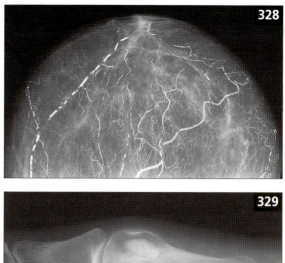

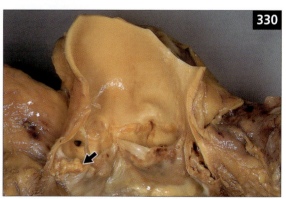

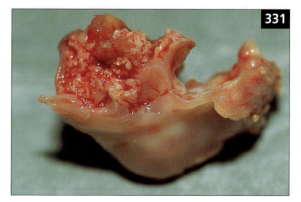

327 Plain X-ray of a long-term dialysis patient showing 'pipe-stem' arterial calcification of both abdominal aorta and iliac arteries.

328 Mammogram showing a skein of 'tram-line' calcifications, with fractures, in the small arteries of the breast in a long-term, diabetic dialysis patient.

329 Hand X-ray showing digital arterial calcification.

330 Postmortem view of calcification of the leaflets of the aortic valve (arrow).

331 Gross destruction of aortic valve by staphylococcal endocarditis and aortic root abscess.

Dialysis (RRT) (*continued*)

Left ventricular changes

Left ventricular changes are virtually ubiquitous in chronic renal failure and dialysis. Left ventricular hypertrophy (LVH) (**332**) can be shown to develop relatively early with declining renal function, and LV mass increases *pari passu* with renal impairment. Concentric LVH is the commonest pattern; some have reported asymmetric LVH in long-term hemodialysis patients. By the time dialysis has started about 50–60% of patients have LVH. This proportion rises rapidly to become 70–90% of longer-term dialysis patients. The reasons are multi-factorial, and include increased large artery stiffening and abnormal hemodynamics, sleep apnea (inducing repeated sympathetic nervous system stimulation during sleep [**333**]), increased systemic BP (including nocturnal hypertension), anemia, fluid overload, the presence of an AV fistula, and hyperparathyroidism. Histologically there has been demonstrated a remarkable degree of intercardiomyocyte fibrosis with relative paucity of capillaries (as well as the expected changes in cardiomyocytes), which most likely contributes to the arrhythmogenicity of dialysis and the incidence of sudden cardiac death in dialysis patients.

LVH is associated with reduced survival on dialysis, even after renal transplantation. Methods to reduce LV mass include daily short-hours hemodialysis, erythropoietin, intravenous alfacalcidol (calcitriol), ACE inhibition, and renal transplantation. After many years of concentric LVH the LV can progressively dilate (**334**) – this is often accompanied by hypotension and 'heart failure' and has a very poor prognosis.

Dialysis-related amyloidosis

Dialysis-related amyloidosis (beta-2-microglobulin amyloidosis) is seen in any subject exposed to dialysis for long enough. Younger subjects typically take 10–20 years to develop this complication, and, as technique longevity on CAPD is much poorer than is the case for HD, it is associated with the latter dialysis modality (but is really only a function of dialysis and time). Beta-2-microglobulin levels are elevated (by lack of renal metabolism and excretion) in CRF and dialysis (indeed it can be used to model larger molecular weight solute dialysis clearances). Its production is stimulated also by the use of less than ideally pure dialysis water in HD, and by the contact of blood with bioincompatible membranes. It may be that the use of hemodiafiltration with these desirable characteristics will delay the onset of this condition. Symptoms usually start in the hands as carpal tunnel syndrome; carpal tunnel release is helpful (and the histology shows amyloid deposits in many but not all cases). If dialysis is prolonged further, recurrence is typical, sometimes with large amyloid deposits (**335**); some patients need repeated carpal tunnel

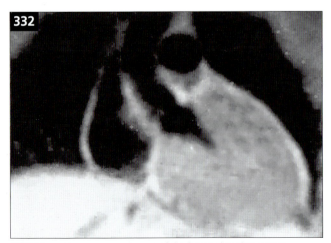

332 Magnetic resonance image of the heart showing severe concentric left ventricular hypertrophy.

333 Output from a sleep apnea study. Oxygen saturation is shown in red in the upper tracing (numerous 'dips' are seen) and pulse rate in blue showing acute rises in heart rate which accompany the falls in oxygen saturation. The yellow symbols on the bottom of the figure show number and severity of apnea episodes.

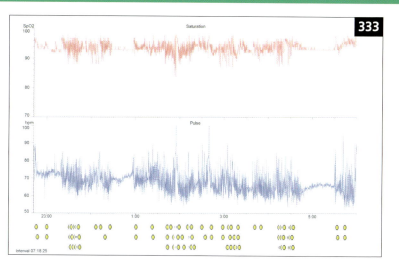

334 Nuclear scintigraphy scan showing (left side) thick wall and tiny LV cavity. Right-sided images show gross LV dilatation.

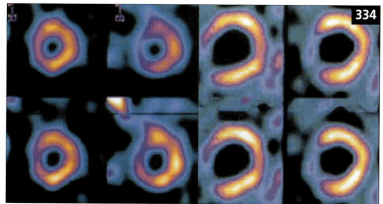

335 Wrist of a long-term dialysis patient. There is already a scar from a previous surgical carpal tunnel release. There is recurrent amyloid tissue (swelling).

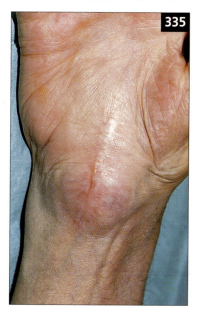

Dialysis (RRT) (*continued*)

surgery. The hands become markedly deformed and the range of finger movement much reduced (**336**). Carpal cysts are seen on plain X-ray (**337, 338**). The shoulders, hips (**339, 340**), and knees can also be affected with severe pain and aching particularly on dialysis; sometimes there can be pathologic fractures. The cervical spine can be involved in an erosive/destructive spondylolisthesis (**341, 342**). Dynamic amyloid scanning can show the amyloid deposits clearly. The deposits in bone are associated with advanced glycation end-product deposition. Regression may occur after successful renal transplantation (and symptomatic relief is obtained quickly on account of the steroids used). There is another rarer form of non-amyloid long-term dialysis small-joint destructive arthropathy (**343**).

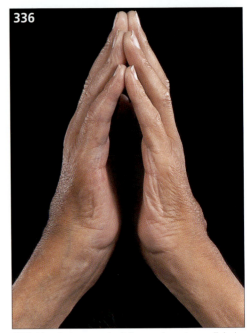

336 Hands (prayer sign) from a long-term dialysis patient with beta-2-microglobulin amyloidosis.

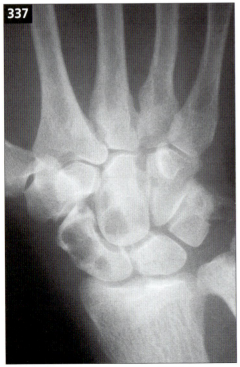

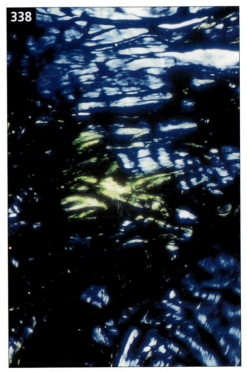

337, 338 Radiologic appearance (**337**) from same patient as **336** with extensive carpal bone cyst formation. Apple-green birefringence (**338**) under cross-polarized light of excised material.

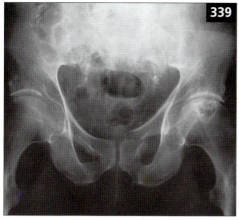

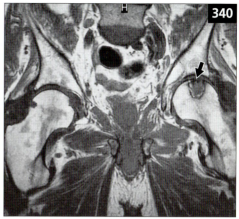

339 Plain X-ray of the pelvis from a patient on dialysis for 26 years and a painful left hip. A large subcapital bone cyst (beta-2-microglobulin amyloid) is seen.

340 MR of the hips from the same patient as **339**. The bone cyst in the left hip is well shown (arrow).

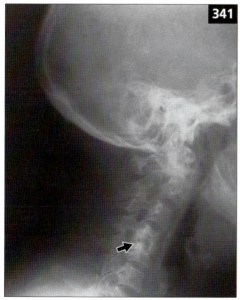

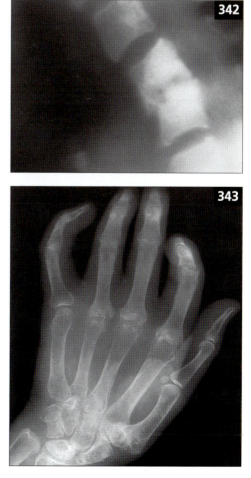

341, 342 Plain cervical spine X-ray (**341**) and cervical vertebral tomography (**342**) showing erosive/destructive cervical spine spondyloarthropathy (arrow).

343 Plain X-ray of the hands showing the rare nonamyloid small-joint destructive arthropathy. Amyloid bone cysts in the carpal bones are also demonstrated.

Dialysis (RRT) (*continued*)

Renal bone disease

Renal bone disease (excluding amyloidosis) is invariable in subjects with chronic uremia or dialysis. It can start with mild chronic renal failure as there is some mild phosphate retention. Hyperparathyroidism, osteomalacia, adynamic bone syndrome (aluminium- and non-aluminium-related), mixed osteodsytrophy and osteopenia are different patterns of skeletal response to chronic uremia, depending on patient population and dialysis treatments. There are characteristic radiologic and histologic (bone biopsy) changes (**344–355**).

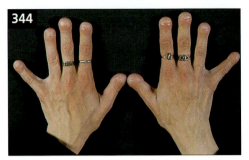

344 Renal pseudo-clubbing indicating terminal digital osteolysis.

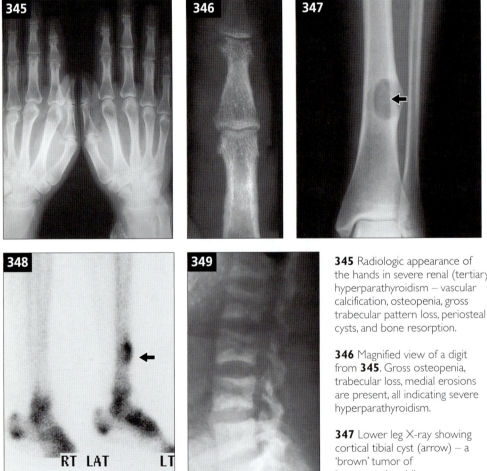

345 Radiologic appearance of the hands in severe renal (tertiary) hyperparathyroidism – vascular calcification, osteopenia, gross trabecular pattern loss, periosteal cysts, and bone resorption.

346 Magnified view of a digit from **345**. Gross osteopenia, trabecular loss, medial erosions are present, all indicating severe hyperparathyroidism.

347 Lower leg X-ray showing cortical tibial cyst (arrow) – a 'brown' tumor of hyperparathyroidism.

348, 349 A bone scan (**348**) showing radio-isotope avidity (arrow) indicating metabolic over-activity, and a lateral X-ray (**349**) of the lumbar spine showing 'rugger-jersey' changes of hyperparathyroidism.

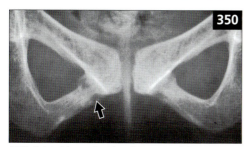

350 Pelvic X-ray showing fractures of the pubic rami (arrow) – Looser's zones, as seen in osteomalacia or the fracturing osteodystrophy caused by skeletal aluminium toxicity.

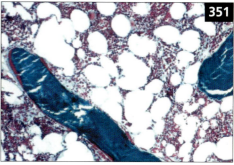

351 Bone biopsy (Girschman trichrome). Normal bone – mineralized osteoid is blue, noncalcified osteoid is red.

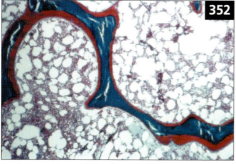

352 Bone biopsy (Girschman trichrome). This shows much increased noncalcified osteoid and is indicative of a mineralization problem, in this case osteomalacia.

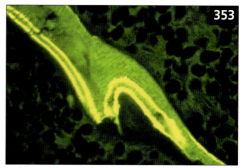

353 Bone biopsy (fluorescence double labeling [tetracycline given as two oral doses 10 days apart]). Gross increase in uptake, and a large gap between the two parallel lines of fluorescence are seen indicating high turn-over bone disease, in this case hyperparathyroidism.

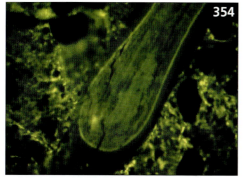

354 Bone biopsy (fluorescence double labeling [tetracycline given as two oral doses 10 days apart]). Virtually no fluoresence, and no double-line is seen. This indicates no bone turnover or adynamic bone syndrome. Few patients are now exposed to aluminium (**355**) – modern causes of adynamic bone are overtreatment of hyperparathyroidism with calcium-containing phosphate binders and vitamin D metabolites.

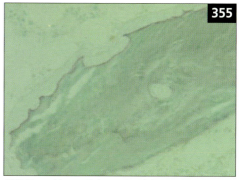

355 Bone biopsy. Faint red staining at the ossification front is aluminium, in this case of aluminium osteodystrophy. Aluminium is one cause of adynamic bone syndrome (giving rise to fracturing microcytic anemia).

Dialysis (RRT) (*continued*)

Parathyroidectomy (PTX)

PTX is required for the majority of patients who have been on dialysis for >10 years. Initial milder forms of hyperparathyroidism can be controlled by prevention or reversal of plasma phosphate elevation, judicious manipulation of dialysate calcium concentrations, and use of vitamin D preparations. If the parathyroid glands become too large, their behavior becomes autonomous and largely refractory to normal physiologic stimuli or pharmacologic manipulation.

Ectopic calcification in skin, muscle, joint or soft tissues, calcific uremic arteriolopathy (calciphylaxis), hypercalcemia, myopathy, tendon rupture, or bone fracture are all indications for surgical parathyroidectomy. Many of the radiologic changes of hyperparathyroidism can reverse/normalize after PTX (**356, 357**). Elevated calcium, phosphate, bone-specific alkaline phosphatase, and PTH are typical. Parathyroid uptake scans show diffusely enlarged overactive glands (**358**) – it is not usually useful to locate glands before a first parathyroidectomy; these glands are often >1 cm^3 when removed. The histology of removed glands usually shows nodular hyperplasia (**359**); very rarely parathyroid carcinoma is found (**360**).

If the patient remains on dialysis for 5 years or more after an initial parathyroidectomy there is a high rate of recurrent/relapsing hyperparathyroidism if a remnant gland was left behind (deliberately or accidentally) or autotransplanted at the initial parathyroidectomy (**361**). Rarely this parathyroid tissue can behave pseudomalignantly as parathymatosis. In these cases preoperative localization of all residual parathyroid tissue in the neck, mediastinum, or limbs is important (it can be done by ultrasound, CT, MR, or by venous-PTH sampling maps).

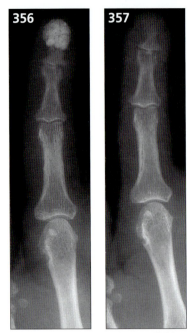

356, 357 Plain X-ray of a digit (**356**) just before surgical parathyroidectomy. Severe changes of hyperparathyroidism can be seen, including ectopic calcification. Six months after the parathyroidectomy (**357**) there has been improvement in many of these abnormal appearances.

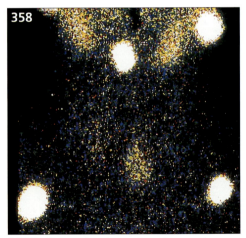

358 Thallium-technetium subtraction scan to visualize abnormal (hypervascular) parathyroid glands. The four white circular areas are the four overactive parathyroid glands in a dialysis patient with hyperparathyroidism.

359 Histology of a parathyroid gland removed at parathyroidectomy. Multiple nodules of hyperplastic parathyroid tissue can be seen (H+E ×30).

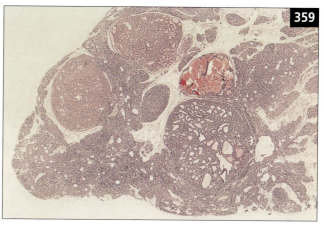

360 Histology of a parathyroid gland removed at parathyroidectomy showing parathyroid carcinoma (islands of malignant cells in vessels in the stroma around the gland). Only 18 cases of this very rare condition have been reported in dialysis patients.

361 A thallium scan showing extensive metabolic activity in a parathyroid autograft in the left deltoid muscle.

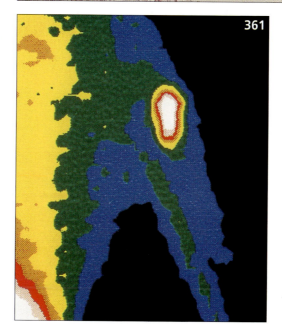

Dialysis (RRT) (*continued*)

Calcific uremic arteriolopathy (CUA, Seyle's calciphylaxis) and calcinosis

CUA and calcinosis are both rare and fascinating conditions. CUA is most commonly seen in patients on dialysis, though can rarely occur in chronic renal failure or after successful renal transplantation.

There is evidence that it is increasing in incidence, though in part this will represent better diagnosis and investigation. Recent evidence about the regulation of calcification (in orthodox and heterodox locations) – which is by means of a wide variety of calcification regulating proteins – has suggested a role for warfarin in inducing metastatic calcifications. This is controversial and obviously has significant implications for dialysis patients. It is clear that in man there are two distinct clinical syndromes (but with uniform histologic findings). The first of these is symmetric ascending acral gangrene, often with painful plaques of skin on the shins (**362, 363**). The second is a destructive necrotic calcifying panniculitis, affecting the pannus typically in poorly-nourished, obese, white, diabetic females (**364**). One of the chief problems, apart from diagnostic suspicion, is the wide differential diagnosis – this must include emboli, cholesterol embolisation syndrome, systemic vasculitis, cryoglobulinemia, cryofibrinogenemia, and systemic oxalosis.

Careful histochemical analysis of a few cases has been performed. A distinctive and previously described small vessel calcification with superimposed endovascular fibrosis was found to be the most common lesion seen in the biopsy material, and was much more frequent than two other lesions proposed to cause the ischemia (thrombosis and global calcific obliteration [**365**]). The calcified stenotic vessels averaged 100 µm in diameter (i.e. small arterioles) and the calcification could also be seen even at capillary level (and clearly therefore adversely affecting tissue oxygenation). Calcification preceded the endovascular fibrosis. Vessels with early endovascular fibroblastic activation were found statistically to be strongly associated with the presence of a giant cell reaction. Proximal locations of necrosis (thighs, buttocks, trunk) carried a more unfavorable prognosis compared to distal locations (calves, forearms, fingers, toes, penis). Diabetics with chronic renal failure had acral gangrene in 61% compared to 34% of the nondiabetic calciphylaxis patients.

In general therapies for this distressing condition are few in number and ineffective. Hyperbaric oxygen therapy (which would counter the severe hypoxia and reduced tissue viability) warrants further study. Parathyroidectomy in the context of obvious biochemical–clinical hyperparathyroidism is associated with a favorable outcome.

Calcinosis refers to the deposition of calcium–phosphate in the skin but without necrosis. It is seen in some patients after prolonged exposure to excessive calcium and especially phosphate. Large, almost tumoral, masses can develop, and strict control of calcium and phosphate balance is mandatory to aid recovery.

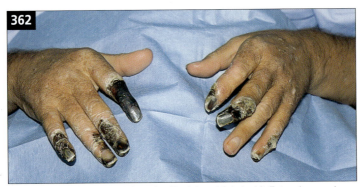

362 Calcific uremic arteriolopathy (Seyle's calciphylaxis). Extensive acral ascending gangrene of the hands.

363 Same patient as **362**. Extensive acral ascending gangrene of the feet.

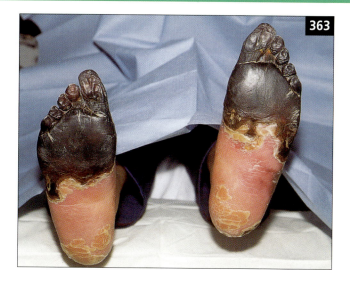

364 Extensive infected gangrene of the pressure areas over the buttocks and thighs.

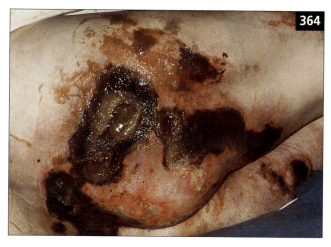

365 Histology of skin shows extensive abnormality including intense medial calcification (arrow) of small arterioles and capillaries, with intense intimal proliferation and thrombosis.

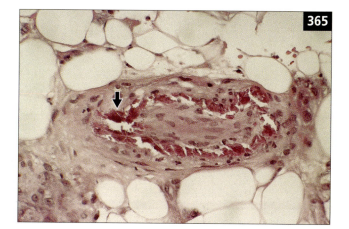

Dialysis (RRT) (*continued*)

Acquired cystic disease of native kidneys

Patients who spend many years in significant renal failure, and particularly on dialysis, develop shrunken native kidneys with large numbers of cortical cysts (**366**). Very rarely these can enlarge massively. These can give rise to retroperitoneal or perirenal hemorrhage (**367**). Renal cell carcinoma can also arise from these cysts – loss of erythropoeitin requirement (due to tumor-related polycythemia) is rare (**368, 369**). Screening for these cysts has been advocated using ultrasound, CT scanning, or MR scanning on a regular basis, but this is not (yet) routine practice. Regression of these cysts can occur slowly after successful renal transplantation.

Diabetic muscle infarction

Diabetic patients with advanced renal impairment, or on dialysis, are prone to this complication. Patients notice muscle weakness (usually thigh) which can be painful accompanied by elevated temperature, inflammatory markers, and muscle enzyme levels (**370**).

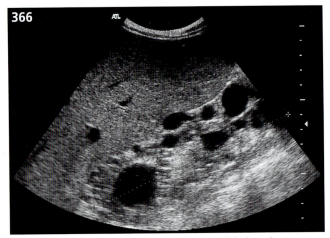

366 Ultrasound of the kidneys in a long-term dialysis patient, showing multiple small cysts uniformly distributed in an otherwise echogenic small kidney.

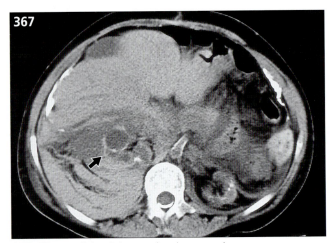

367 CT scan of the abdomen showing a massive retroperitoneal/pararenal hematoma (arrow) in a long-term dialysis patient. The tiny native kidney is hard to distinguish.

368 Renal cell carcinoma arising from acquired renal cystic disease. CT scan of the abdomen to investigate weight loss and reduced erythropoetin requirements in a long-term dialysis patient, showing a right renal mass (and biopsy needle).

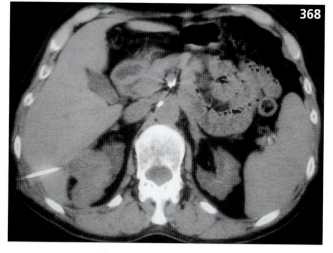

369 Nephrectomy specimen from the same patient as **368** showing multiple small cortical cysts and large renal cell carcinoma.

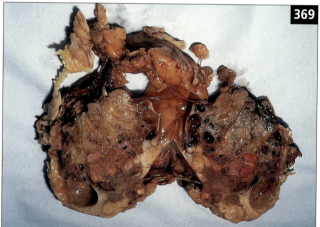

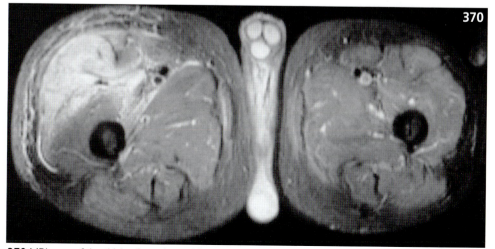

370 MRI scan of the thigh of a patient with acute diabetic muscle infarction. Increased muscle signal is due to increased water content.

Dialysis (RRT) (*continued*)

Infections
Renal patients are much more prone to infections, and sepsis is a major cause of morbidity and mortality on dialysis. Renal patients, especially using dialysis cannulae, repeatedly get bacteremias. These are a major cause of endocarditis. In addition, there is a greatly increased incidence of staphylococcal (and other organism) vertebral diskitis (**371**, **372**), which require long-term antibiotics and often surgery. Renal patients are also more prone to *Clostridium difficile* diarrhea and pseudomembranous colitis (**373**, **374**). Tuberculosis is also more common in both hemodialysis and also peritoneal dialysis patients.

Malignancy on dialysis
There is a small but significant increase in the incidence of solid-organ and bone-marrow tumors in dialysis patients.

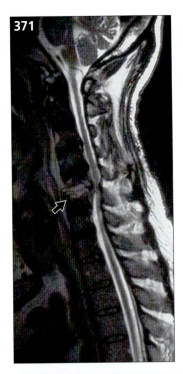

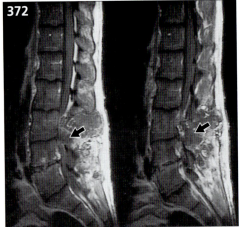

372 CT scan of the lumbar vertebrae. A paravertebral abscess (arrows) and facet joint infection are shown (this was staphylococcal in origin).

371 MRI scan of the cervical vertebrae. A paravertebral abscess and cervical diskitis are shown (arrow). This was 'sterile' on aspiration, biopsy, and culture but settled on antibiotics.

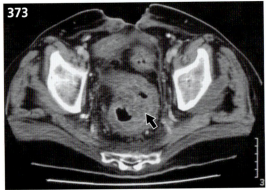

373, 374 CT scan of the abdomen (**373**) with bowel and intravenous contrast showing the grossly thickened/edematous rectal wall (arrow), and sigmoidoscopic appearances (**374**) showing gross edema and pseudomembrane formation.

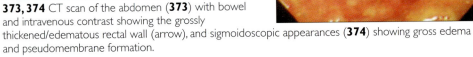

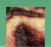

Chapter Twelve

Renal transplantation

- **Introduction**

- **Causes of graft dysfunction**

- **Renal allograft histology**

- **Vascular and urologic complications of renal transplantation**

- **Other complications**

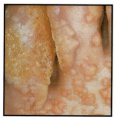
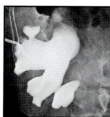
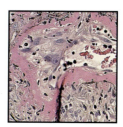
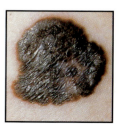

Introduction

Renal transplantation is now the treatment of choice for most patients with end-stage renal failure. Transplantation has been shown to improve long-term survival and quality of life compared to patients who remain on dialysis. Combined kidney–pancreas transplantation is the optimal treatment for selected type 1 diabetics.

Patient and graft survival at one year is excellent, although graft loss from chronic allograft nephropathy remains a major problem.

However, graft survival is improving; the projected half-lives of grafts performed in 1995 in the USA were 21.6 years for recipients of living donor grafts, and 13.8 years for cadaveric grafts. The improvements are due to increased experience of transplant teams, better HLA matching, and newer immunosuppressive agents and antiviral drugs.

In this chapter, we will highlight some of the clinical problems after renal transplantation.

Causes of graft dysfunction

When renal allograft dysfunction occurs it is necessary to find the cause. Common reasons are hypovolemia, acute pyelonephritis, drug toxicity, acute or chronic rejection, recurrent or *de novo* glomerular disease, or vascular and uro-logic complications. Imaging is initially performed by ultrasound which will detect transplant hydronephrosis or a lymphocele. Subsequently, renal biopsy is often essential to define cause of graft dysfunction and guide therapy.

Renal allograft histology

Following renal transplantation, there are three major periods: delayed graft function, early dysfunction, and late dysfunction.

DELAYED GRAFT FUNCTION
This refers to failure of the graft to function from the moment that the clamps are removed from the renal vessels and may last for a very variable period, usually only for a few hours or days, but on occasion for several weeks, with eventual onset of adequate function. Management of the patient during this period requires regular renal biopsies to exclude rejection.

Delayed graft function may be associated with a variety of processes, and these include:
- Acute tubular necrosis.
- Accidents to the vascular or ureteric anastomosis.
- Perfusion injury.
- Hyperacute rejection.

Acute tubular necrosis
The pathologic appearances of acute tubular necrosis vary greatly in degree, from incipient infarction to mild and focal attenuation of tubular epithelial cells (Chapter 10). This process may be accompanied by a variable degree of interstitial edema but is not associated with cellular infiltration. There is a notoriously poor correlation between the pathologic changes and the degree of dysfunction, and it is unreliable to predict the speed of recovery from the severity of the appearances. Sometimes it may take weeks for the onset of renal function. High levels of calcineurin inhibitors may prolong the process.

Accidents to the vascular or ureteric anastomosis
There are no reliable pathologic features to diagnose or exclude these possibilities. Thrombosis of the main renal artery will give rise to nonhemorrhagic infarction, whereas thrombosis of the main renal vein will cause hemorrhagic infarction.

Perfusion injury

There may be obvious damage to endothelial cells, or in extreme cases changes in the wall of arteries indistinguishable from fibrinoid necrosis. These appearances may also be seen in non-heart beating donors, and can cause the pathologist a serious diagnostic dilemma in making a distinction from vascular rejection. The diagnosis may only be revealed by time, in that recovery is unlikely in vascular rejection, but function may ensue after perfusion injury. Perfusion injury may be accompanied by a fall in the platelet count, which may help to distinguish these conditions.

Hyperacute rejection

Hyperacute rejection is seen very occasionally (**375, 376**). It is caused by the presence of circulating antibodies from previous sensitization of the recipient, which react with antigens that are present in the donor kidney. These are most commonly ABO or HLA Class I antigens. A negative cross-match between donor lymphocytes and recipient serum guards against such an event. However, accidents can occur – e.g. if the cross-match sample predates sensitization caused by a blood transfusion. A situation mimicking hyperacute rejection can be caused by cold-reacting IgM antibodies. This can be avoided by ensuring that the donor organ is at body temperature before the clamps are removed from the vascular anastomosis.

The pathologic appearances of hyperacute rejection are of platelet thrombi in the microcirculation, with margination of polymorphs, proceeding to hemorrhage and necrosis.

EARLY GRAFT DYSFUNCTION

This may be defined as the onset of dysfunction after a period of adequate function, and may start within a few days to a few months after transplantation. It is in this period that acute rejection becomes one of the most important possibilities to exclude, because early and effective treatment will be necessary to limit the degree of irreversible damage and give the greatest chance of prolonged good function.

During this period, therefore, the possible diagnoses include:
- Acute tubular necrosis.
- Acute cellular rejection.
- Accidents to the vascular or ureteric anastomoses.
- Calcineurin inhibitor toxicity.
- Acute vascular rejection.
- Infection, including pyelonephritis, cytomegalovirus, polyoma virus.

Acute cellular rejection

Acute cellular rejection may be seen as early as the fifth day after transplantation, but is more commonly seen after one week. It becomes decreasingly common as each week passes, but may occasionally be seen years after transplantation, usually

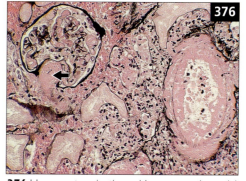

375 Photograph of a kidney that has undergone hyperacute rejection.

376 Hyperacute rejection, with transmural arterial infarction, fibrin thrombus in afferent arteriole (arrow), death of tubules, and peritubular hemorrhage. Light microscopy (MS ×250).

Renal allograft histology (*continued*)

in association with noncompliance with medication. Cellular rejection accounts for approximately 90% of acute rejection episodes.

The microscopic features are very similar to an acute tubulointerstitial nephritis of any cause, for example drug sensitivity. There is a diffuse interstitial cellular infiltrate composed mainly of T-lymphocytes and macrophages, and these cells characteristically infiltrate the tubular epithelium, causing destruction of the epithelial cells and the tubular basement membrane (**377**, **378**). There may be associated hemorrhage and edema. The earliest cellular infiltration is seen around the interlobular veins. Natural killer cells and plasma cells are only seen in small numbers. Occasionally there are significant numbers of eosinophils. It is important to remember that the renal medulla is not usually involved, even in severe cellular rejection. This means that if the biopsy core does not include cortex, acute cellular rejection cannot be reliably excluded.

Acute vascular rejection (379–381)
There are a variety of factors involved in this process. These include circulating antibodies directed at various sites such as the endothelium or the muscle cells of the vessel wall, or the direct cytotoxic effect of specific T-lymphocytes. It is sometimes possible to demonstrate the presence of anti-HLA antibodies in the recipient's serum; however, vascular rejection may be seen in the absence of recognizable antibodies.

From a practical point of view it is possible to distinguish a process that mainly affects capillary size vessels, as opposed to larger vessels such as arterioles and arteries. In rejection of the kidney, veins do not appear to have a significant role other than allowing lymphoid cells access to the renal parenchyma. When capillary-sized vessels are involved, the result is interstitial hemorrhage due to damage to peritubular capillaries. When large vessels are principally involved, they may show a variety of changes such as:
- Endothelial cell swelling or necrosis which can result in thrombosis.
- Margination and infiltration by mononuclear cells (intimal arteritis).
- Fibrinoid necrosis of the vessel wall.
- Mucoid intimal proliferation (similar to that seen in HUS).

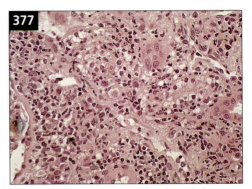

377 Acute cellular rejection showing tubules intimately mixed with mononuclear cells. It is difficult to detect tubulitis without a basement membrane stain. Light microscopy (H+E ×250).

Early recognition of vascular rejection may be aided by staining of the biopsy with antibodies to C4d. Positivity will be seen in peritubular capillaries. This apperance occurs before the more serious features listed above, and will allow appropriate treatment to be started sooner.

Calcineurin inhibitor toxicity
The appearances in cyclosporine (cyclosporin) toxicity are identical to those in tacrolimus toxicity. The following three features, although not specific to calcineurin inhibitor toxicity, if taken with the appropriate clinical picture, i.e. graft dysfunction with high drug levels, will help in making the diagnosis:
- The presence of hyaline lesions in arterioles (**382**). The interpretation of these appearances has to be taken with caution because many donors are hypertensive and it is difficult to be certain that such changes did not come with the kidney from the donor.
- Isometric vacuolation in tubular epithelium (**383**). This is the presence of multiple small clear vacuoles of similar size. This appearance is only infrequently present, and is often only limited to occasional tubules, but when present is a very useful diagnostic feature.
- Peritubular and glomerular capillary thrombi, although not specific, are a useful feature.

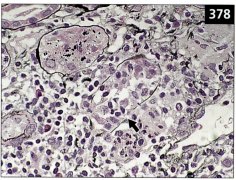

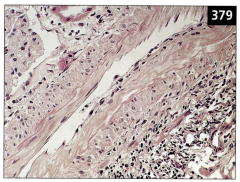

378 Acute cellular rejection showing mono-nuclear cells infiltrating into the tubular epithelium (tubulitis) with destruction of the basement membrane (arrow). Light microscopy (MS x400).

379 Acute vascular rejection. Interlobular artery showing intimal arteritis. Light microscopy (H+E x250).

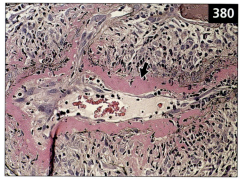

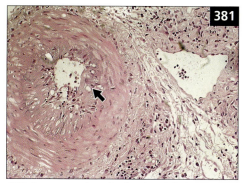

380 Acute vascular rejection. Interlobular artery showing intimal arteritis and fibrinoid necrosis of the vessel wall (arrow). Light microscopy (H+E x250).

381 Acute vascular rejection. Interlobular artery showing mucoid intimal proliferation (arrow). Light microscopy (H+E x250).

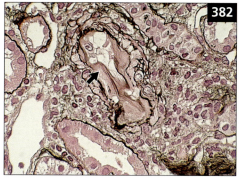

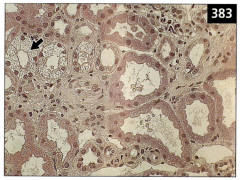

382 Calcineurin inhibitor toxicity. Arteriole showing hyaline change (arrow). Light microscopy (MS x400).

383 Calcineurin inhibitor toxicity. Tubules from a child on cyclosporine (cyclosporin) for a liver transplant showing isometric vacuolation (arrow). Light microscopy (H+E x250).

Renal allograft histology (*continued*)

Infection

The main infective processes affecting the renal transplant are:

- Acute pyelonephritis.
- Cytomegalovirus infection.
- Polyoma viruses including BK and JC.

Dysfunction may be attributable directly to the infective process or as a result of the infection inducing an episode of acute rejection.

The diagnosis of acute pyelonephritis will usually be made on account of pain, pyrexia, and pyuria. Occasionally the presence of large numbers of polymorph casts within tubules in the renal biopsy can be the first indication of infection.

Cytomegalovirus infection is sometimes associated with graft dysfunction without rejection. A biopsy taken under these circumstances may occasionally show the characteristic inclusions in tubular epithelial cells or glomeruli (**384**).

More recently infection with polyoma viruses, including BK and JC, have been recognized. These infections are associated with a gradual decline in graft function often many months after transplantation. It is recognized that these infections are more common with intensive immunosuppression. The initial poor prognosis has improved with the strategy of reducing immunosuppression and use of the antiviral drug cidofovir. The biopsy shows chronic tubular damage associated with characteristic nuclear and cytoplasmic changes in the tubular epithelium (**385**). Urine cytology will show 'decoy cells' consisting of sloughed-off renal tubular cells with inclusion bodies (**386**).

LATE GRAFT DYSFUNCTION

This clinical period extends from several months to years after transplantation. Some of the conditions encountered during this period are listed below:

- Chronic rejection.
- Chronic allograft nephropathy.
- Chronic calcineurin inhibitor toxicity.
- Recurrent glomerular disease.
- *De novo* glomerular disease.
- Post-transplant lymphoproliferative disorder.

Chronic rejection

This term is an attempt to link an etiologic process with a pathologic appearance which includes chronic glomerular, interstitial, and vascular damage. These appearances may be arrived at by a wide variety of pathologic processes which may include: recurrent episodes of cellular or vascular rejection, reflux nephropathy, or graft ischemia. It is not generally possible to distinguish between these etiologies by the pathologic appearances.

Chronic allograft nephropathy

It is more appropriate to consider all of the chronic changes that occur in the transplant under this heading, rather than chronic rejection, and to include the specific glomerular appearances of transplant glomerulopathy.

Transplant glomerulopathy (**387, 388**) is generally associated with the onset of significant proteinuria, which may reach nephrotic levels. There are characteristic pathologic appearances which include glomerular hypercellularity, endothelial swelling, and double-contouring of the glomerular capillary walls. Immunohistochemistry usually shows little immunoglobulin or complement deposition, although sometimes there may be capillary wall localization of IgM, making distinction from membranoproliferative glomerulonephritis difficult. Electron microscopy will show an electron-lucent subendothelial zone in allograft glomerulopathy, whereas electron-dense deposits are expected in membranoproliferative lesions.

Chronic calcineurin inhibitor toxicity

Chronic toxicity causes tubular damage and interstitial fibrosis. Sometimes the pattern of damage gives rise to bands of fibrous scarring alternating with relatively well-preserved tubules. This is known as striped fibrosis.

Recurrent and *de novo* glomerular disease

Some glomerular diseases are particularly prone to recur in grafts and cause graft loss, especially focal and segmental glomerulosclerosis, membranoproliferative glomerulonephritis, and familial hemolytic–uremic syndrome. IgA nephropathy frequently recurs but rarely causes early graft loss.

Any form of glomerular disease may occur *de novo* in a renal graft. The presenting symptoms will be the same as in native kidneys. The pathologic appearances may be more difficult to assign because of the potential similarities between allograft glomerulopathy and membranoproliferative glomerulopathy, HUS, and accelerated phase hypertension.

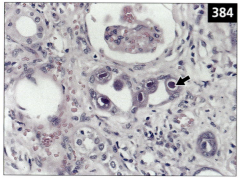

384 CMV. Tubular cells contain 'owl-eyes' intranuclear inclusions (arrow). Light microscopy (H+E x250).

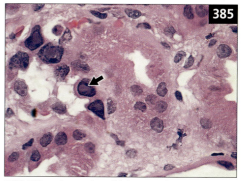

385 BK nephropathy with intranuclear inclusions within renal tubular cells (arrow). Light microscopy (H+E x400).

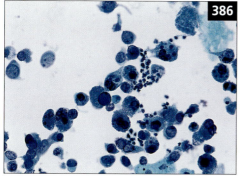

386 BK nephropathy. Urinary cytology showing decoy cells.

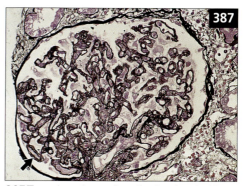

387 Transplant glomerulopathy showing double-contouring of the capillary walls (arrow). Light microscopy (MS x400).

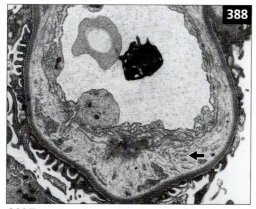

388 Transplant glomerulopathy with wide sub-endothelial electron-lucent zone (arrow). Electron microscopy (x5000).

Renal allograft histology (*continued*)

Post-transplant lymphoproliferative disorder

There is a spectrum of proliferative disorders of lymphoid cells that may occur in transplant recipients. Generally these are B-cells and are of host origin, and are most commonly associated with Epstein–Barr virus. At one end of this spectrum, there is a polyclonal B-cell proliferation that presents as an infectious monucleosis type of illness, and will respond to reduction or withdrawal of immunosuppression, while at the other there is an aggressive monoclonal proliferation that behaves like a high-grade lymphoma, requiring treatment with chemotherapy and anti-B-cell monoclonal antibodies.

About half of patients with PTLD present with extranodal disease, and about one-quarter show involvement of the graft kidney, which may result in dysfunction. Distinction from cellular rejection may require immunopheno-typing (**389, 390**). Rejection is associated with T-cell infiltration while PTLD is usually associated with B-cells. It is also possible to demonstrate EBV in a proportion of the cells in PTLD by *in situ* hybridization.

Banff classification of renal allograft pathology

This is a continually evolving international consensus amongst pathologists who are involved with the interpretation of renal allograft biopsies. The purpose is to standardize the interpretation of allograft biopsies in order to guide therapy and give an objective end point for clinical trials.

Table 17 The Banff 97 schema
Normal
Antibody-mediated rejection
Borderline changes, 'suspicious of acute rejection'. This shows mild tubulitis, but no vascular changes
Acute rejection Type: IA Significant interstitial mononuclear infiltration, but only moderate tubulitis IB Significant interstitial mononuclear infiltration, with severe tubulitis IIA Mild to moderate intimal arteritis. IIB Severe intimal arteritis III Transmural arteritis and/or arterial fibrinoid change
Chronic allograft nephropathy Grade I: mild interstitial fibrosis and tubular atrophy Grade II: moderate interstitial fibrosis and tubular atrophy Grade III: severe interstitial fibrosis and tubular atrophy
Changes not considered to be due to rejection

The Banff 97 schema includes six diagnostic categories, which are presented in a simplified form in *Table 17*.

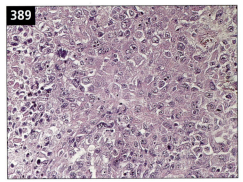

389 Post-transplant lymphoproliferative disease. High power view showing pleomorphic lymphoblastic infiltrate in an aggressive PTLD. Light microscopy (H+E ×400).

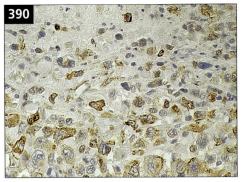

390 The same case as **389** showing cells staining positively with antibody to EBV Light microscopy (immunoperoxidase ×400).

Vascular and urologic complications of renal transplantation

LYMPHOCELE

Definition
Lymphoceles are collections of lymph around the renal transplant.

Epidemiology and etiology
Up to 50% of renal allograft may have lymphoceles detectable on ultrasound. Most resolve spontaneously, and intervention is required only in the minority.

Pathogenesis
Most lymphoceles arise from leakage of unligated iliac vessel lymphatics of the recipient, rather than from the graft itself. The incidence of clinically significant lymphoceles appears higher in patients receiving sirolimus therapy, because sirolimus slows wound healing.

Clinical history and physical examination
Most lymphoceles are clinically silent. Larger lymphoceles can present with swelling around the graft, leg swelling, worsening renal function, and deep vein thrombosis. Most present within 2 weeks to 6 months after transplantation, with a peak incidence at 6 weeks.

Differential diagnosis
The principal differential diagnosis is a pyogenic collection. There is usually a raised white cell count and CRP; aspiration will confirm infection.

Investigations (391)
Ultrasound is the easiest method of imaging. Lymphoceles are characteristically homogeneous and lie between the kidney and the bladder.

Prognosis
Small lymphoceles resolve spontaneously, whereas larger ones require intervention. Complications include infection of the collection and deep venous thrombosis.

Management
Intervention usually initially involves percutaneous drainage which may need repeating. However, lymph may continue to drain and surgery may be required. The technique termed fenestration involves creating a window between the collection and the peritoneum.

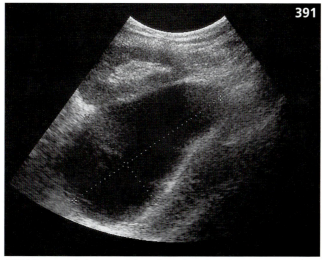

391 Ultrasound demonstrating a large lymphocele.

Vascular and urologic complications of renal transplantation (*continued*)

RENAL ARTERY STENOSIS

Definition
Whereas renal artery or vein thrombosis (**31, 32**) are the commonest causes of immediate graft loss after transplantation, renal artery stenosis is an important late complication.

Epidemiology and etiology
The incidence varies in different series (1–12%) and partly depends on the rigour of the screening policy adopted by individual units. The causes are probably multifactorial involving atheroma in the donor vessels, technical errors, chronic immune damage, and CMV infection. The peak time of presentation is 3 months to 2 years after transplantation.

Clinical history
Patients may present with a rising creatinine or with worsening hypertension. A substantial rise in creatinine after initiation of ACE inhibitors is a characteristic presentation. Flash pulmonary edema may also occur. A bruit may be audible.

Differential diagnosis
A critical stenosis of the proximal iliac vessels may mimic renal artery stenosis.

Investigations
Noninvasive methods of screening include power Doppler ultrasound (**392, 393**) and magnetic resonance angiography (**394**). These have the advantage of avoiding nephrotoxic contrast. Digital subtraction angiography remains the gold standard, and if doubt remains the pressure gradient across the stenosis can be measured (>20mmHg [2.7 kPa] is significant).

Prognosis
If a critical stenosis is left untreated the graft function and hypertension will usually deteriorate. Re-stenosis may occur postangioplasty.

Management
Percutaneous transluminal renal angioplasty is the treatment of choice for most functionally significant lesions. There is a small risk of arterial occlusion with graft loss. Re-stenosis should be suspected clinically, and power Doppler can be used as a sensitive screening technique.

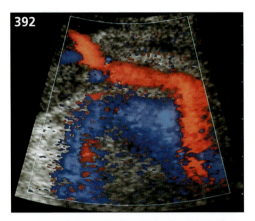

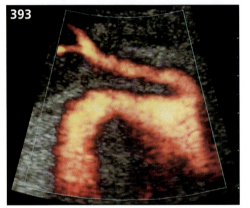

392, 393 Color Doppler ultrasound (**392**) and power Doppler ultrasound (**393**) of a normal renal transplant.

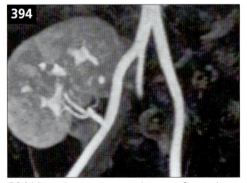

394 Magnetic resonance angiogram of a renal transplant (normal study).

URETERAL OBSTRUCTION
Definition
Ureteral obstruction is an important cause of impaired or deteriorating graft function.

Epidemiology and etiology
It may occur early or late after transplantation. It may be caused by extrinsic compression of the ureter by a lymphocele or hematoma, or by a hematoma or calculus within the lumen. Ischemia may also cause stricturing of the ureter.

Clinical history
The transplant kidney is not innervated and therefore obstruction is usually painless. There is usually a rise in creatinine.

Investigations
Ultrasound will in most cases show hydronephrosis. Antegrade pyelogram will demonstrate the site of obstruction as well as relieving obstruction (**395**). Furosemide (frusemide) renography can help to distinguish between true obstruction and a large floppy pelvicalyceal collecting system.

Prognosis
This depends on the cause of the obstruction. Ischemic strictures need surgical intervention.

Management
Obstruction can be temporarily relieved by insertion of a nephrostomy or stent. Urinary tract infections should be treated. Surgery may be required for definitive treatment.

Other complications

CARDIOVASCULAR
Cardiovascular disease is the commonest cause of death after renal transplantation, and is a major target of intervention. Coronary artery disease and left ventricular hypertrophy are prevalent in patients with chronic renal failure (Chapter 11). The hypertension and dyslipidemia induced by steroids and calcineurin inhibitors are risk factors for accelerating atherosclerosis. Aggressive control of blood pressure and lipids is vital in the management of post-transplant patients.

MUSCULOSKELETAL
Bone disease is a major complication of renal transplantation, especially in postmenopausal woman who already may have pre-existing osteoporosis. Patients will have pre-existing renal bone disease from their chronic renal failure (Chapter 11). After transplantation patients may lose 10–15% of their bone density in the first few months due to initial immobilization and high doses of steroids used. Thereafter bone density stabilizes or even rises. The incidence of vertebral and hip fractures is greatly increased. Modern immunosuppressive regimens involve minimizing corticosteroids. Bisphosphonates may be useful in preventing post-transplant osteoporosis.

Avascular necrosis of the hip (**396**) was a particularly common complication in the pre-cyclosporine (cyclosporin) era because larger doses of corticosteroids were given. Treatment requires hip replacement.

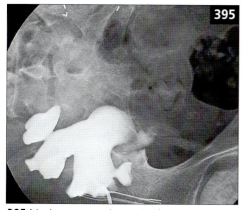

395 Nephrostogram demonstrating hydronephrosis in a renal transplant.

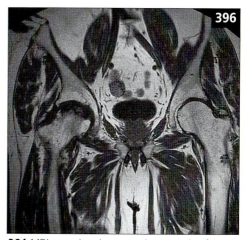

396 MRI scan showing avascular necrosis of the hips.

Other complications (*continued*)

NEUROLOGIC
Immunosuppression can lead to unusual central nervous system infections by organisms such as *Cryptococcus, Aspergillus, Nocardia*, and *Listeria*. Calcineurin inhibitors cause a tremor in a dose-related fashion. Rarely, they can cause reversible posterior leucoencephalopathy syndrome: this may present with blindness, fits, and decreased conscious level (**397, 398**).

INFECTION
Renal transplant recipients are susceptible to pyogenic bacterial infections in the first few days and weeks after transplantation. This is because of the immunosuppression caused by the uremic state as well as the immunosuppressive drugs used. Host defences are breached by central lines, urinary catheters, and sometimes by contaminated organs. Wound, pulmonary, and urinary infections are common.

Thereafter opportunistic infections become a more serious problem. Calcineurin inhibitors selectively inhibit T-cell function, and so the infections that are controlled by cell-mediated immunity tend to predominate (as in HIV infection). Viruses, mycobacteria, protozoa, and certain fungi are important potential pathogens in transplant recipients.

Viruses
Viral pathogens that definitely cause disease in transplant recipients are listed in *Table 18*.

Cytomegalovirus (CMV)
This is probably the most important viral pathogen affecting renal transplant recipients. It may be either transmitted by the graft or reactivated in the recipient by immunosuppression. The most severe infections tend to occur in patients who have a primary infection at the time of transplantation. Without antiviral prophylaxis, symptoms and signs of infection begin 4–8 weeks after transplantation. Usually there is fever, leucopenia, and thrombocytopenia. Tissue-invasive disease can affect the esophagus, colon, liver, lungs, and retina (**397**). Various techniques have been available to monitor CMV infection, but direct antigen testing (DAT) and CMV PCR are the most widely used. Prophylaxis is now given to high-

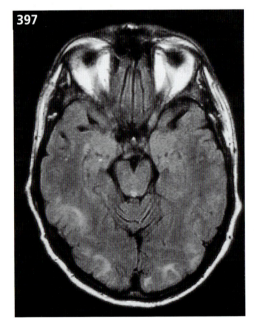

397 MRI scan in a man who developed reversible blindness secondary to cyclosporine (cyclosporin) – 'reversible posterior leucoencephalopathy syndrome'. The scan shows lesions in the occipital cortex.

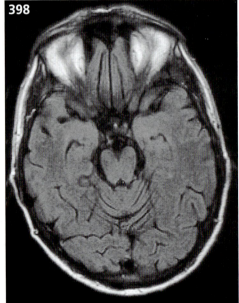

398 A follow-up scan in the same patient as **397** after a full recovery following discontinuation of cyclosporine (cyclosporin).

risk recipients by using ganciclovir or valacyclovir (valaciclovir). Treatment involves reducing immunosuppression and intravenous ganciclovir. A rare complication of prolonged ganciclovir usage is the development of ganciclovir-resistant mutant strains.

Table 18 Viral pathogens that definitely cause disease in transplant recipients

Virus	Clinical manifestation
Herpes simplex	Cold sore (**399**)
Herpes zoster	Chickenpox/shingles (**400**)
Cytomegalovirus	Fever, leucopenia, pneumonitis, hepatitis, colitis, retinitis
Epstein–Barr virus	Post-transplant lymphoproliferative disease
Human herpes virus-8	Kaposi's sarcoma
Hepatitis B and C	Hepatitis, cirrhosis
HIV	Immune deficiency
Polyomaviruses	
BK	Interstitial nephritis, ureteric stenosis, cystitis
JC	Progressive multifocal leucoencephalopathy
Papillomavirus	Warts, squamous cell carcinoma

399 Herpes simplex infection on the lip.

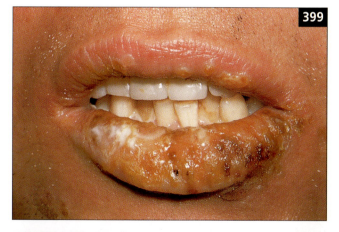

400 Herpes zoster infection on the buttock.

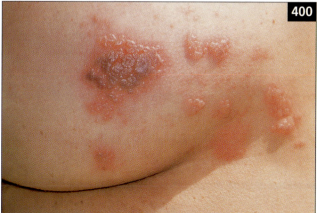

Other complications (*continued*)

Opportunistic pathogens

Important nonviral opportunistic pathogens are listed below:

- Bacteria: *Legionella*, *Nocardia* (**401**), *Mycobacteria*.
- Fungi: *Pneumocystis* (**402**), *Candida*, *Aspergillus* (**403**), *Cryptococcus*, *Mucormycosis*, *Coccidiomycosis* and histoplasmosis in endemic areas.
- Parasitic: *Strongyloides*, toxoplasmosis.

NEOPLASIA

There is an increased incidence of certain malignancies in the transplant population due to the long-term effects of immunosuppressive drugs reducing tumor surveillance, activating oncogenic viruses, and increasing production of proproliferative cytokines such as TGF-β. Lymphomas (**399, 404**), cervical carcinoma, and skin malignancies are particularly found in the transplant population.

Skin tumors

Skin tumors are the commonest malignancy in transplant recipients. They are particularly prevalent in areas of the world where sun exposure is great. In a study from Queensland in Australia, the cumulative incidence of basal cell and/or squamous cell carcinoma rose from 7% at 1 year to 45% at 11 years and 70% at 20 years following transplantation. Squamous cell carcinomas (**405**) occur with a greater incidence than basal carcinoma which is a reverse of the incidence in nonimmunosuppressed individuals. Squamous cell carcinoma tend to be multiple, recur and metastasize more readily than in the normal population. In the Australian population malignant melanoma (**406**) was four times more prevalent in the transplant population.

Kaposi's sarcoma (**407**) is found most commonly in transplant patients of Arabic, African, or Mediterranean origin. Human herpesvirus-8 is implicated in its pathogenesis. The tumors may appear on the skin as purple macules or in the mouth, respiratory, or gastrointestinal tract. They may regress after reduction in immunosuppression and may respond to local radiotherapy.

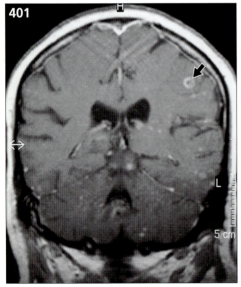

401 MRI brain scan in a renal transplant patient with cerebral nocardiosis (arrow).

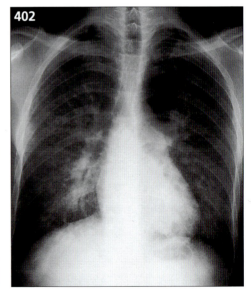

402 CXR of a patient with *Pneumocystis carinii* pneumonia.

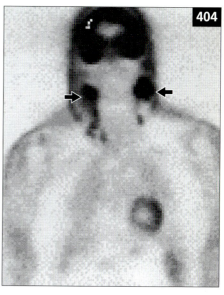

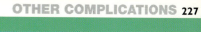

403 CT scan demonstrating an aspergilloma in a renal transplant patient.

404 PET scan demonstrating increased uptake in the cervical glands (arrows) in a patient with post-transplant lymphoproliferative disease.

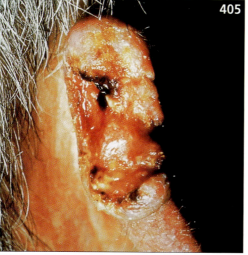

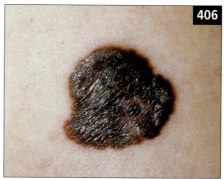

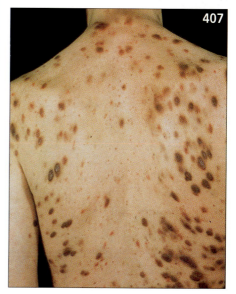

405 Squamous cell carcinoma on the ear.

406 Malignant melanoma.

407 Multiple cutaneous Kaposi sarcoma lesions.

Other complications (*continued*)

COSMETIC

Immunosuppressive drugs can cause undesirable cosmetic side-effects.

Steroids cause an increase in appetite and a change in body fat distribution causing 'moon-like' facies, truncal obesity, and striae formation. Steroids also induce acne mainly over the face, upper trunk, and upper arms (**408**).

Cyclosporine (cyclosporin) causes marked gingival hyperplasia (**409**) especially when used in conjunction with the antihypertensive drugs nifedipine or amlodipine. The gum hypertrophy may be very severe, but will regress if the offending drugs are discontinued. Cyclosporine (cyclosporin) may also cause severe hypertrichosis within the first 6 months of treatment (**410**). Tacrolimus does not cause either of these side-effects.

Viral warts (**411**) are very common in transplant recipients. They correlate with the degree of sun exposure and duration of immunosuppression. They may be multiple and difficult to distinguish from squamous cell carcinomas. They may cause much cosmetic surgery. Treatment involves minimizing immunosuppression, cryosurgery, and topical or systemic retinoids.

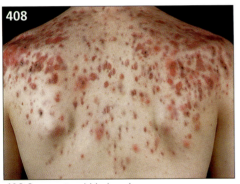

408 Severe steroid-induced acne.

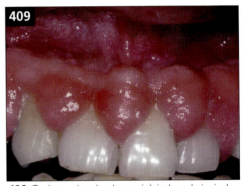

409 Cyclosporine (cyclosporin)-induced gingival hyperplasia.

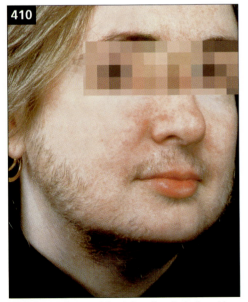

410 Severe hypertrichosis in a female induced by cyclosporin (ciclosporin).

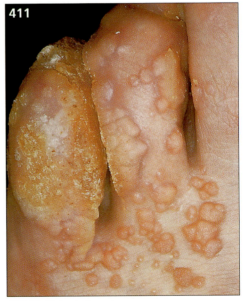

411 Multiple viral warts.

Index